Dedication

This book was written for my mom...

"Thanks for taking my advice and changing your life."

YSWLY

Table of Contents

Foreword

I have spent over 20 years as a private trainer, health club operator and health club owner. I have always had the dream of permanently changing someone's life. The kind of change that is so amazing that the person remembers you for the rest of their life.

With a little luck and over 1000 hours of research, I have finally achieved my dream.

I would like to share with you a miracle...

A Personal Note from the Author

I was born Dec 8, 1967, in W. St. Paul, Minnesota. I was raised to believe in God and to help your neighbor whenever possible. I graduated from junior college and then went to college at Cal State Fullerton. After college, I entered the health club industry where I proceeded to work for the next 21 years. I opened seven health clubs for three different health club chains. I held every position imaginable in the health club field: janitor, front desk, trainer, certified personal trainer, salesperson, assistant manager, manager, and part owner of multiple health clubs. I am definitely qualified as an expert in the field of health clubs and fitness.

As a kid growing up in Minnesota, I was extremely skinny. The doctor advised my parents to feed me white bread and Miracle Whip to "fatten me up." It didn't seem to work. I remained a less-than-normal weight through my teen years. At the age of 19 I started to work in a health club and began to body build. My body was very receptive to the "body building supplements" that I was taking, and I ended up packing on some noticeable muscle. One day on a trip to Tijuana, Mexico, I was hit by a car while walking and was incapacitated for several months. During this time I continued eating like a body builder while lying on the couch like a couch potato. I ended up packing on some unwanted fat that haunted me for the next 21 years.

As a health club owner/operator, I was constantly pressured to lose the extra weight and slim down. I tried every diet along with exercise. **I worked out one hour per day (average) for 15 years straight.** (Some days I would miss my workouts, other days I would work out for multiple hours.) The workouts were great for my cardiovascular system and to maintain my muscle tone, but ineffective in the long run for permanent weight loss.

I would watch people kill themselves everyday working out to lose weight, knowing the entire time that as soon as they stopped exercising at that intensity they would gain the weight back along with additional weight. The trainers would flat out say to their clients that _**70-80% of their results would be due to their diet.**_ The private trainers would joke that clients were paying them thousands of dollars for "temporary results."

I was caught up in a whirlwind. I knew firsthand the pressure and humiliation my clients received every day! They say that the best salespeople can put themselves in the client's shoes, and I am living proof of this. For years and years I was one of the top salespeople at one of the biggest (open all hours) health club chains in the United States, and I was overweight.

Like some of my fellow health club employees, I always felt guilty selling people "the health club lie." I spent many nights going home and drinking away my guilt. I would convince myself that, "at least I was giving the people the opportunity to get in shape." I knew deep down inside this was a lie, and I spent years feeling bad about myself as a person. I felt like I was not only lying to people, but also stealing money from those I sold memberships to. I prayed that someday I would have the opportunity to make amends and make it right.

One day my prayers were answered.

I stumbled across the Hcg weight loss program. I discovered that this program was very popular and effective in the 1950's and 1960's and just recently it was experiencing a revival.

I spent four hours a day, every day (except Christmas and Thanksgiving) for the next year studying Hcg weight loss. I communicated via telephone, email and mail to dozens of doctors, pharmacists, naturalists, herbalists, and to a chat site of over 1500 past and present Hcg dieters that were scattered all over the world. My goal was to invent a new way to do the Hcg program making it more available to more people. My goal was twofold - to invent a way to take Hcg without painful injections, and to make the Hcg program affordable to every person possible.

On day 366, I put my plan into action and started on my journey...

I was working at a different (open all hours) health club chain.   The first thing I did was to tell my two co-workers, Lucas and Justin, what I was about to do. I then told my two roommates, Mike and Marty, what I was about to do. I knew in my heart I was about to undergo an amazing change, and I didn't want my friends to think that I was losing weight because I was sick or abusing drugs. My buddies were definitely skeptical, but they had seen me intensely study the program for the last year. They all gave their support.

I continued on my journey…

46 days later, I was exactly 50 pounds lighter!

During those 46 days, the "bad feelings of guilt" I had experienced while selling health club memberships in my younger years started to re-emerge. I was still selling the "health club lie." I was losing weight at an amazing rate while doing absolutely no exercise at all! I was telling people that my results were due to the training staff and the use of the cardiovascular equipment. I felt so guilty that I started to do abdominal exercises with the clients of the trainers. Every day I felt more and more guilty. I was getting ten times the results of the clients that were being trained, and I wasn't exercising at all! Every day I dreaded going to work to sell memberships. A few days later the owner was forced to sell the health club and my days in the health club industry were over.

I proceeded to coach 50 of my closest family members and friends on the weight loss program I had designed. The people ranged in age from 18 years old up to 68 years old. To my amazement, all 50 people lost incredible weight. The women averaged 0.5 pound weight loss per day over six weeks and the men averaged 1.0 pound per day weight loss over six weeks. My 67-year-old mother lost 80 pounds in 93 days! My best friend ended up losing 136 pounds over an 8-month period. During that period, he only did the diet five out of the eight months. As I write this book, he has been on a regular diet for over four months and is still within five pounds of his lowest weight. He has no stretch marks and no baggy skin. He has easily added 20 years to his life and subtracted 10 years from his appearance.

Several of my former health club workers have done this program, and they all agree that **this is the only way they have ever discovered to permanently lose weight and restore their metabolism to normal!**

In 22 years of fitness, health and diet experience, this is the only permanent, non-surgical solution to weight loss that I have ever seen!

The days of "suffering on a diet and looking tired and haggard on a diet" are finally over!

Many of my friends have urged me to write this book. So, here it is…

Introduction

As I am writing this book, my mother is waging a brutal battle against cancer. I have seen firsthand the way "cures" for all kinds of aliments are being hidden from the common person.

I believe that everyone has an inalienable right to live the healthiest and disease-free life possible. It is a shame that some individuals and companies will let people suffer and die just so they can make an extra buck.

My goal is to reveal to you a weight loss miracle that will shed those extra pounds, reset your metabolism, and make you feel fantastic and alive. I want this to be available to everyone!!! Right now, a 4-6 week program can be completed for roughly $100.

Almost every one of my clients/friends who have undertaken my program has saved more money on their grocery bill than what they invested on the Hcg Weight Loss program!

An old friend said it best when he said, "Mark, this is the investment of all time, and in the end it didn't end up costing me a dime!"

"I have never heard of or encountered an individual that did not lose noticeable weight on this program. I have communicated with thousands of individuals that have participated in this program".

Mark Pirkl, Author

This is it! The real deal! Please take advantage of this program while you can!

The Difference between This Program and the Programs Offered at the Weight Loss Clinics

My goal is to provide you with a simple and easy program to follow. <u>I have strived to make the program as "dummy proof" and as inexpensive as possible!</u> I have modified the original protocol so this program can be done without having to take injections.

The Appendix of this book contains the Doctor's original protocol that I have based my program on. The changes I have made to the original protocol are designed to maximize your results and to simplify the process.

The original protocol works perfectly, and if you prefer to stick strictly to the doctor's original protocol, I encourage you to do so.

Many weight loss clinics have had some sort of Hcg weight loss program for the last 10-20 years. Most people have never heard of the program because the clinics don't advertise the program. They want to stay off the FDA's radar. Many people who complete this program are no longer on their lifetime prescription of different medications. Drug companies don't like people getting healthy, because when people get healthy, they often no longer need prescription drugs.

Most clinics that offer Hcg programs charge anywhere from $750-$1,500 a month. In addition, the client often has to undergo their program twice as long to get the same results as they would on this program. Most of the clinics could make the weight disappear twice as fast as they do, but clinics stretch the treatment out... not for health reasons, but to make more money from the client.

On a clinic program, clients have to fit a daily visit into their lifestyle. They have to experience <u>multiple painful injections every week</u>! The client isn't free to travel or go on a vacation. They must stay within driving distance of the clinic so they can receive their injections each week.

The benefits of this program, compared to most of the clinics that offer the Hcg weight loss program, include;

- *COMPLETE PRIVACY*

- *THE SAME OR BETTER RESULTS IN ALMOST ½ THE TIME*

- *A COST OF LESS THAN 1/5 TH OF WHAT MANY CLINICS CHARGE*

- *NO PAINFUL INJECTIONS!*

- *FREEDOM FROM HAVING TO SCHEDULE MULTIPLE APPOINTMENTS EACH WEEK*

- *THE ABILITY TO LEAVE THE AREA AND TRAVEL ON VACATION OR BUSINESS*

- *THE FREEDOM TO SPEED UP, SLOW DOWN, OR PUT THE PROGRAM ON HOLD FOR ANY REASON*

- *THE COMFORT AND SAFETY OF NEVER HAVING TO LEAVE YOUR HOME*

Q&A

Q - My friends have done the Hcg weight protocol through a weight loss clinic and have had to do painful injections every day. I am terrified of needles! Is there any way to do this program without having to take injections?

A - Unlike most weight loss clinics, this guide will show you how to take the supplement sublingually/orally (painlessly held and absorbed by holding it in your mouth under your tongue).

Q - If I undergo a VLCD (very low calorie diet), won't I get extremely hungry?

A - The supplement causes the body to mobilize stored fat and use it as energy. When the fat is mobilized it not only keeps most clients feeling satiated, it also releases vitamins and minerals that are stored in the fat. This combination not only makes most clients feel and look better, it also increases the energy level for most people.

Q - Will I need a doctor's prescription to be able to purchase and take the supplement?

A - This guide will show you how to obtain approval and purchase the supplement online by filling out a simple medical questionnaire.

Q - My friends that have done this program through different weight loss clinics have had to spend about $800 - $1,500 monthly for this program. How much is this going to cost me?

A - This guide will show you how you can do the program for a fraction of what the weight loss clinics charge. *Note: Almost every client has positively commented on how the money they saved on their monthly food bill covered most of the cost of their program. In some cases, the money saved by the reduction in food consumption was enough to cover their investment in the program.*

Q - Are there any adverse side effects?

A - The program has very few side effects. Some clients experience mild to medium hunger the first week to 10 days of their program. **Some clients that didn't take their potassium supplements everyday experienced severe muscle cramps**! Headaches are common the first three days of the program, due to withdrawal from carbohydrates. Clients have experienced mild hair loss that reversed itself after they completed the program. There have been cases where clients have experienced rashes on the fatty areas of their bodies for a day or two. This is due to the fact that toxins are being eliminated through the skin as the body burns fat.

Q - What are some positive side effects?

A - Most clients experience rapid weight loss, increased energy levels, loss of hunger daily, improved skin tone, a reduction in blood pressure, reduction in body aches and pains, better sleep, reduction/elimination in snoring, healthier hair and nails. Some clients have reported having their sleep apnea, diabetes, and/or their high blood pressure eliminated. Clients have also reported a reduction or elimination of psoriasis.

Q - Once I stop the program will I gain the weight back?

A - The program helps the body reset its hypothalamus gland and return the metabolism back to normal. Most clients that complete the program and then return to eating a "healthy normal diet," keep the weight off for more than 10 years (this is based on phone interviews and email conversations with dieters that participated in this program in the 1950's and 1960's).

Q - How long does the program take?

A – Average programs are 23 - 60 days long with a 6-week maintenance program afterwards. Men average a one pound weight loss per day. Women average a 0.5 pound weight loss per day.

Q – Should I expect to lose weight every day?

A - You won't lose weight every day, and some days you may actually gain weight due to water retention.

Q – Do I need to eat special foods on this program?

A - Please refer to the manuscript "Pounds and Inches. The food involved is readily available at almost every grocery store.

Q - I only want to lose 5 or 6 pounds, can I do the program?

A - This program is only recommended to clients who want to lose 10 or more pounds of fat.

Q - Can I work out on this program?

A - Light exercise is highly recommended (example-golf, long walks, playing with your children, gardening). Heavy weight lifting, aerobic exercise, and strenuous exercise are not allowed.

Q - What if I don't want to exercise?

A - The program's average weight loss is based on averages for clients **who did not exercise**. Clients who exercised lightly while on the program lost more than the average weight loss.

Q - Can I drink alcohol during the program?

A – Alcohol is not allowed (as it contains empty calories). Please refer to the manuscript "Pounds and Inches."

Q – Does everyone lose weight on this program?

A - I have never had or know of an individual that followed the program completely and did not lose noticeable weight.

Q - What will I need to buy in addition to the supplement and groceries?

A - You will need to have a good quality digital bathroom scale, digital food scale, a bottle of daily whole food supplements, and a bottle of 99mg potassium tablets.

Medical Disclaimer

This book is designed to "guide" you (help you everyday) to stick to an Hcg diet protocol that has been in existence for over forty years and is taken from a manuscript called "Pounds and Inches A New Approach to Obesity" by Dr. A.T.W.Simeons M.D. The protocol calls for a specific 500 calorie a day diet along with doses of Hcg that are to be taken every day.

This protocol has never been approved by the FDA for weight loss or for the treatment or diagnosis of any other medical condition.

Although there are little or almost no know side effects with this protocol, each individual will react differently to the diet and the author can't offer any medical advice whatsoever. Although the author has had great success "guiding" his friends on this protocol, **he has no medical training and no formal Hcg medical training.** This book is designed to simplify the Hcg diet in addition to guiding you in making sure you stick strictly to the diet in Dr A.T.W. Simeons' protocol "Pounds and Inches A New Approach to Obesity." It will also show you how and where to obtain the food and Hcg needed to be a success.

The author strongly advises you to consult your physician before starting the program (or any diet program) and **if at any time you don't feel well, you are also advised to immediately stop the program until you consult with a physician. You are free to discontinue the diet program at any time for any reason.**

You need to understand that although women average a 0.5 pound a day loss on average (on a 26 day or longer protocol) and that men average a 1.0 pound per day (on a 26 day or longer protocol) that results may vary from individual to individual. There is a chance you may not lose any weight at all.

The author has communicated via phone and Internet to thousands of people regarding the Hcg diet. They include actual Hcg weight loss participants, physicians, and pharmacists. **He has never encountered an individual who has participated in the program and followed the protocol and not lost noticeable weight.**

The author is not qualified to and refuses to offer any medical advice at any time. **Information in this book must NOT be construed as medical advice.** The author cannot be held liable for any physical, psychological, or emotional reactions that may result from this diet, whether the reactions are positive or negative.

The information contained in this book is not intended to diagnose, treat, or cure any medical condition. The information is not designed to be a substitute for any medical treatment, evaluation, or diagnosis.

An Overview of the Program

For the first four days (96 hours) of the program, you will gorge on high fat foods until you are "stuffed" everyday. During these first four days you will also be taking the Hcg sublingually every day.

After day four (96 hours), you will discontinue gorging on fat and start on the 500-calorie per day diet **(VLCD/very low calorie diet).** You will remain on the VLCD for **a minimum of 23 more days**. Your weight loss goal and actual weight loss will determine how long you will stay on the VLCD.

Once it is determined that you have reached your final day of the VLCD, you will record your **last dosage weight (LDW)** and discontinue the use of the Hcg. You will continue the VLCD for 3 more days (72 more hours) while the Hcg leaves your system.

For the next three (3) weeks you will increase your food intake to at least 1,500 calories per day. The "average" person will be consuming somewhere around 1,500 - 3,500 calories a day. During these three (3) weeks you will slowly add the following fats to your diet: vegetable, animal, dairy. Examples of these fats are guacamole, cheese, olive oil, coconut oil, meat, dairy, etc. During these three (3) weeks you must keep your weight within 2-3 pounds of your LDW.

For the following three (3) weeks you start to slowly add sugar, starches, and carbohydrates to your diet. At the same time, you will continue to keep your weight within 2-3 pounds of your LDW.

Once you have finished the VLCD and 6-week maintenance period, your body weight set point will be set to your new body weight, and your metabolism should be reset to function normally.

You can now enjoy your new metabolism and a whole new life!

What Most People Experience During and After the Program

The Good:

- A gorging feast the first four days of the program

- **An almost zero net cost for this program** because you are saving more money on your food bill than what you invest on this program

- A remarkable drop in weight after 1-3 days on the VLCD

- The reduction or complete **elimination of snoring**

- No hunger or almost no hunger during the entire program

- An amazing increase in energy

- Extreme weight loss without experiencing additional "stretch marks" or "loose and baggy skin" when you are finished

- **Extreme weight loss without having to exercise**

- A more youthful appearance

- A whole body detoxification

- Amazing reduction in the "hard to lose" fat areas of your body

- **Extreme weight loss without having to eat foods you don't like or don't normally eat**

- Many people experience a noticeable decrease in alcohol, nicotine, or drug cravings

- A more attractive complexion

- Complete privacy and anonymity

- The elimination of many weight-related medical problems, and the elimination of the drug prescriptions that they have been taking to treat those problems

- A redistribution of remaining body fat that puts their body back into normal proportions

- Most people experience an "improved or better singing voice." Professional singers often enjoy drastic weight loss while still retaining their singing voice.

- Healthier looking hair, skin, and nails

- A metabolism that is now restored to normal

- A decrease in high blood pressure and an increase in stamina

The Bad:

- **Extreme muscle cramps for people who let their potassium levels drop too low**

- Resistance from your family and friends because you are only consuming 500 calories a day and they don't understand how the protocol works

- Some people experience mild headaches the first 2-3 days on the diet

- Some people feel sick the first few days of the VLCD (very low calorie diet) due to Candida die-off and toxins being eliminated from their system

- No alcohol is allowed after day one of the VLCD

- Occasional and short bouts of slightly blurry vision

- Many doctors that have been in practice less than 30 years will tell you they don't know anything about the program or have never heard of it

- Your need to use the bathroom to relieve yourself might increase twice or three times as much as normal while you are on the program

- Some people experience itchy or blotchy rash areas that last for a day or two on their abnormally fat areas (this is believed to be due to an excess of toxins being flushed out of those areas)

- Trouble staying warm at first, due to the dramatic loss in body fat

- Most people have to purchase a whole new wardrobe because most of their clothes have become way too big to wear

- A loss of anywhere from 1-3 days of results for each time you even slightly cheat on your diet

- Most people have an extremely tough time not cheating on the diet if they are undergoing the diet during the holiday season

- Resistance training/weight lifting or heavy or strenuous exercise is not allowed while on this diet

- Diet sodas are not recommended while on this diet

- Many people experience constipation and need to use a laxative or some other bowel movement stimulator while on this program

- A minimum of one gallon of water is recommended to be consumed _every day_ of the diet

- You will be required to write down _everything_ you eat _every day_ you are on the program

- Little or no tolerance to alcohol once the program is completed. Some people become violently drunk/ill after consuming their "usual" amount of alcohol

- An increase in fertility/the ability to become pregnant for women that are still able to become pregnant and are not taking birth control

- A feeling of fatigue for some people who don't eat the recommended amount of protein each day

The Ugly:

- Some people experience strong and even severe emotional flashbacks. This is due to the release of toxins that were stored in the fat cells during past emotional or traumatic events

- Some people (recovering alcoholics/smokers) experience the taste of nicotine or alcohol due to those stored toxins being released from the fat cells

- A very small amount of women have experienced noticeable hair loss while on the program (Hair volume returned to normal after the program ended, in all the cases we know of)

Before You Start

THINGS TO <u>SERIOUSLY CONSIDER</u> BEFORE STARTING THE PROGRAM:

- Do you have any special events coming up that will interfere with your program (vacations, work meetings, holidays, travel plans, surgeries) and make it difficult to stick with the program?
- Are you committed to achieving your goals?
- Are you going to get "road blocked" by roommates or friends and family?
- Can you avoid consuming alcohol during the program?
- Are you going to have time to do the program (pre-purchase the food needed and prepare your meals before leaving home for the day)?
- Can you purchase the items needed **before** you start your program?
- You will be drinking more water than usual (for most people) and having to use the restroom quite often. Will your daily activities allow you use of the restroom during the day?
- Will you be able to weigh yourself first thing **each morning** and write down what you eat each day?
- Do you need approval from your doctor due to existing health problems and medication that you are taking?
- Are you ready for **drastic change** and to start a whole new life?
- Are you emotionally attached to your current body size?

It is also recommended that you read the manuscript "Pounds and Inches A New Approach to Obesity" by Dr. A.T.W. Simeons, located in the Appendix of this book. You will find your results will be much greater if you understand why you are doing what you are doing while on this protocol. Dr. A.T.W. Simeons' manuscript does a great job of explaining how and why the protocol works.

What You Need to Get Started

(Do not start the program unless or until you have EVERY ONE of the mandatory items!)

Mandatory Items:

- A quality, digital scale that measures in 0.2 to 0.5 pound increments (You must be able to step on the scale three (3) times consecutively within a 2-minute period and get the same reading on the scale each time. If you can't get the same reading three times in a row, then your scale cannot be used for the program.). Most people purchase the "Thinner" brand scale for about $40 from Bed Bath & Beyond, or 3D Bed and Bath.
- A quality food scale that will measure food in grams and ounces.
- 30 or more days worth of Hcg supplement, mixing ingredients, and storage vial
- A refrigerator to store your Hcg supplement once it is mixed
- A week's worth of protein (chicken, fish, lean beef) and at least a four (4) day supply of vegetables/fruits
- Freezer ziplock storage bags for the meat
- A whole food supplement (whole food tablets such as *Superfoods* and *Megafoods*. A whole food supplement is similar to a multi-vitamin and can be found in the multi-vitamin section of your local health food store)
- Himalayan, Celtic, or Mediterranean Sea Salt
- Some type of easy cooking device for your meat (Flavorwave turbo cooker is highly recommended. Most people have some kind of George Forman cooker or something similar)
- Apple cider vinegar, Braggs liquid aminos and liquid Stevia sweetener.
- A bottle of 99mg potassium tablets

Suggested Items (may or may not be needed during your program):

- A food chopper or grinder
- MSG free seasoning for the protein you will be eating
- Hair/skin products that do not contain fat (for those clients that are hyper-sensitive to fat absorption)
- A carbohydrate free laxative product (smooth move tea, oxygenated magnesium, enema kit, etc.)
- Warm clothes

Ordering Your Hcg and Other Items Needed

Ready...   Set...   Go...

This program is not designed for or tested on individuals under the age of 18. If you are under 18 years of age, you must get a doctor's approval and supervision to participate in the HCG program.

My goal is to give you the most current information on how and where to order Hcg and which companies offer it for the cheapest price, fastest delivery, and best customer service. It is often difficult to find one company that encompasses all three criteria. I will also include as much contact information for each company as possible.

Due to the increase in popularity of the Hcg diet you may find that companies are temporarily out of stock of the product. **It is important that you have your complete cycle of Hcg in your possession before you start your program!**

Ordering Hcg

It's time to order your Hcg. My favorite site currently is: www.alldaychemist.com.

Some of the websites will send you Hcg whether you have a doctor's prescription or not. *I always advise to get a doctor's prescription for your Hcg.* I would hate to have to live with the thought that someone had some rare body type that reacted negatively to Hcg and that they went and ordered it without a doctor's prescription anyway. Although I have never heard of or communicated with anyone that could not safely take Hcg, I am sure that there is some person who may react negatively to Hcg.

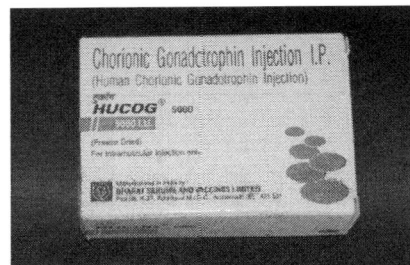

When you order your Hcg, there is a good chance that it will be shipped from a pharmacy in a different country.

I have had many dieters express concern that they were worried that the Hcg they were receiving was not "real" or not as potent because it came from a foreign country (this concern is especially prevalent within the weight lifting/body building community that has often ordered steroids costing hundreds of dollars each only to find out that they received a fake or counterfeit product). To the best of my knowledge, all pharmaceutical companies manufacture their products under the same guidelines. This means that all products are manufactured the same and contain the same ingredients. It would not be worth the time or money for a company to counterfeit a product as inexpensive as Hcg. So to sum it up, think of the different brands of Hcg the same as you would aspirin. Bayer aspirin and generic aspirin are going to be manufactured the same and contain the same ingredients and have the same effect. A 5000 iu vial of Hcg is going to be manufactured the same, contain the same ingredients, and be the same strength from one company to the next.

I have had several friends try HOMEOPATHIC Hcg, some have had great success and some have had no results at all. At the current time, I can't recommend HOMEOPATHIC

28

Hcg because there is no way to know that what you are getting is real. When you order pharmaceutical Hcg, you know that it is real.

Before you order, you will need to try to calculate how much Hcg you will need. A huge mistake that many Hcg dieters make is that they **do not** order all their Hcg at one time. They order a partial order to try it out, and then they run out before their next order arrives. You need to know that this program has worked for thousands and thousands of people. **I have never communicated with or have heard of a person who has gone through the program and not lost noticeable weight/inches.**

With this in mind, ***I would not recommend this program unless you are willing to order a complete cycle of Hcg before you start!***

Calculating your order

#1 – How much weight are you trying to lose? If you are trying to lose less than 10 pounds, this program is not for you.

#2 – For women, divide the number of pounds you want to lose by the number 7. For men, divide the number of pounds you want to lose by 14.

#3 - Your answer will be the number of vials/ampoules of Hcg that you need to order before starting the program. For example, a female and a male both want to lose 28 pounds. The female would need to divide 28 by 7 to come up with 4 ampoules/vials of Hcg. The male would want to take 28 divided by 14 which equals 2 ampoules/vials of Hcg.

If the number calculates out to be between two (whole) numbers, you want to round up to the higher number. For example, if your answer calculates out to be 3.19, you will need to round up to next higher number, 4. So, you would want to order 4 vials/ampoules of Hcg.

Here are the sites to order from (as of late 2009):

www.alldaychemist.com – by far the most inexpensive and fastest delivery. Many people have difficulty ordering from this site. If you do not have a Visa credit card, it seems more difficult to get your order through.

www.reliablerxpharmacy.com – (213) 291-0788 – almost identical in price and delivery as alldaychemist.com. Often it will have the greatest variety of Hcg brands available for sale.

www.axroids.com – the second fastest in delivery and easy to place an order.

www.drugdelivery.ca – the most popular order site. This site is the easiest to place an order with, but has the longest delivery time.

If you have trouble with the above websites, I recommend contacting a great group of folks who have been invaluable to me. They are a group of Hcg dieters that belong to a chat group *HcgDieters@yahoogroups.com*. These folks are wonderful, very helpful and very understanding. They have been the answer to many of my questions in the past, and they will most likely give you the most current website of the best company to order from.

Once again, I would not recommend this program unless you are willing to order a complete cycle of Hcg before you start!

Mixing Supplies

For every 15 days you plan on being on the program you will want to have the following:

- One (1) amber colored 30 ml vacuum sealed vial with a rubber stopper

- Three (3) 22-gauge 1.5 inch needles with 3 ml/cc syringes (Don't worry, the needles <u>are not</u> for injections.)

- One 10 ml/cc mixing syringe with 22-gauge needle

Needles can be removed or replaced on syringes by simply twisting them on or off the syringe. Syringes may be reused (used for more than 15 days) and needles should be discarded after five (5) days.

Reminder: the needles are for mixing the product, storing, and removing it from the vacuum sealed container. ***YOU WILL NOT BE RECEIVING/TAKING INJECTIONS UNDER THIS PROTOCOL.*** This protocol is designed to be taken sublingually (<u>painlessly</u> held and absorbed under your tongue).

Here are the sites to order mixing supplies:

www.gpzservices.com - I order from gpzservices.com. They are extremely reliable and inexpensive. See below for ordering instructions.

www.researchsupply.net

www.syringesupplies.com

http:/catalog.bd.com

www.qualitymedicalsupplies.com

www.Hcgsupplies.com

GPZ Services, Inc. ordering instructions:

The following are instructions on how to do an order from www.gpzservices.com:

- First go to the website gpzservices.com. You will get to a home page with a menu on the left side of page

- Click on the section for "products"

- Scroll down until you find **Vials – Presealed** and click on it *(picture)*

- Click on the word **Amber.**

- Scroll down to **30 ML Presealed Vial (Amber)** and order 1 bottle for every 15 days you plan on being on the VLCD diet and then click on "Add To Cart"

- When it shows your shopping cart, click on the Continue Shopping box.

- Click on the section for "products"

- Scroll down to **Syringe with Needle** and click on it (picture)

- Click on **3 CC Syringe with Needle** (picture)

- ➢ Scroll down to **3 CC syringe with Needle, 22G X 1.5"** (picture)

- ➢ Order three (3) – for every 15 days you plan on being on the **VLCD** and click on Add To Cart (once again, these syringes and needles <u>are not</u> being purchased for self injection)

- ➢ When it shows your shopping cart, click on the Continue Shopping Box

- ➢ Go back to the menu and click on the section for "products"

- ➢ Scroll down to **Syringe Only** and click on it (picture)

- ➢ Scroll down to **Syringe only, 10 CC** and order one and click on Add To Cart

- ➢ Click on the Check Out box and complete your order

Waiting for Your Hcg

While you are waiting for your Hcg, it is highly recommended that you do a Candida cleanse (intestinal cleanse). This will help with cravings when you start your program. Candida cleanse is available in both 15-day and 30-day packages at most health food stores.

You can plan on your Hcg taking anywhere from 14 – 40 days to arrive at your address. Most pharmaceutical companies will send you a notice and a tracking number once your product has shipped. Many companies also offer an express shipping option for an extra charge.

Once your product has been shipped, it will have to clear through U.S. Customs before it arrives at your home. Customs can take one to three weeks to forward your order. Orders, which contain more than 3-months worth of many different medicines, will often get "held up" in Customs or even confiscated. Please keep this in mind when ordering your Hcg. Most companies will replace your order if it gets confiscated while going through Customs.

If you are having the product delivered during the hot summer months, please be aware that the Hcg should never be stored above room temperature. If you are not going to be home the day of delivery, and it is hot outside, you might want to make arrangements for a neighbor to bring your package in out of the hot sun. I have had clients who left their Hcg in their postal delivery box for several days during the hot summer. When they went to use the Hcg, they discovered the "above room" temperature had ruined the potency of their Hcg.

If you are not home when your delivery arrives, it is a common occurrence for your Hcg to be held at the post office or by the shipping company. The post office usually holds your delivery in a cool dry area until you come in and sign for it or they ship it back.

If they were ordered the same day, your mixing supplies (syringe, needles, and storage container) will usually arrive just before your Hcg arrives.

Yippee!!! The Hcg has Finally Arrived

Attention ladies: You should not start this program if you are within five (5) days from the start or finish of your menstrual cycle. You also want to do your best to avoid the finish of your Hcg program coinciding with the start of your monthly cycle.

The following is taken from Dr. Simeon's manuscript "pounds and inches" located in the Appendix of this book:

(Remember, you will not be taking injections with this program!)

Menstruation

During menstruation no injections are given, but the diet is continued and causes no hardship; **yet as soon as the menstruation is over, the patients become extremely hungry unless the injections are resumed at once.** It is very impressive to see the suffering of a woman who has continued her diet for a day or two beyond the end of the period without coming for her injection and then to hear the next day that all hunger ceased within a few hours after the injection and to see her once again content, florid and cheerful. While on the question of menstruation it must he added that in teenaged girls the period may in some rare cases be delayed and exceptionally stop altogether. If then later this is artificially induced some weight may be regained.

Just a reminder of what to consider before starting your program:

- Do you have any special events coming up which will interfere with your program (vacations, work meetings, holidays, travel plans, surgeries) and make it difficult to stick with the program?
- Are you committed to achieving your goals?
- Are you going to get "road blocked" by roommates or friends and family?

- Can you avoid consuming alcohol during the program?
- Are you going to have time to do the program (pre-purchase the food needed and prepare your meals before leaving home for the day)?
- Can you purchase the items needed **before** you start your program?
- Will your daily activities allow you use of the restroom during the day? You will be drinking more water than usual (for most people) and having to use the restroom quite often.
- Will you be able to weigh yourself first thing **each morning** and write down what you eat each day?
- Do you need approval/prescription from your doctor due to existing health problems and medication that you are taking?

If you think nothing from the above list is going to interfere with your program, then it's time to mix your Hcg.

Mixing Your Hcg

Supplies

Before you mix your Hcg, you will need to have all the following items together in one place:

One (1) - 30ml amber sealed vial

One (1) – one ounce (shot-sized) bottle of **clear** flavored vodka

Distilled water – a gallon costs about a dollar and is available at most grocery stores.

One (1) – 10 cc/ml syringe and one – 3 cc/ml syringe

One (1) – 22, 23 or 25 gauge needle that is at least 1 ½ inches long

One (1) – 5000 iu vial/ampoule of Hcg

One (1) – six inch (or larger) square piece of tinfoil

Mixing Instructions

REMINDER: At no point will you be taking injections. The needle is for mixing purposes only!

Step 1 – Open a single box of your Hcg.

Inside you should find two ampoules or one ampoule and one vial. An ampoule has a sealed glass container made completely of glass. It **will not** have a metal, plastic, or rubber top. **It will resemble a miniature glass bowling pin.**

If your box has a vial in it, the vial will look like a miniature jar with a colored plastic cap on it. Almost every box of Hcg should or will have an ampoule or vial of mixing liquid with it. It is very important that you identify which one is the Hcg ampoule/vial and which one is the mixing liquid. The mixing liquid will be liquid and will most likely be labeled "sodium chloride for injection" or "bacteriostatic water for injection".

IMPORTANT - Hcg has recently started being manufactured and shipped in liquid form. If you package has 2 vials/ampoules of liquid, You will know which one is Hcg because it will be labeled **_Human Chorionic Gonadotrophin._**

If your box of Hcg has 2 ampoules in it, then we need to practice opening an ampoule...

We are going to use the ampoule of liquid to "practice on" <u>before</u> we try opening the ampoule of Hcg.
Make sure the practice ampoule has mixing liquid in it and <u>not</u> Hcg!

Take the ampoule and score around the narrowest part of its "neck" using a paring or small sharp knife. I use a small quarter sized Dremmel sanding/cut off wheel that you can purchase at the hardware section of Walmart or at most Hardware stores.

When scoring the neck, try not to cut through the neck or break the bottle. Once the neck has been scored all the way around, you want to hold the

ampoule by the "body" of the ampoule with your first and second finger. You want the top of the ampoule to be pointed toward the ceiling. (You should be holding the ampoule like you would hold a cigarette lighter). While holding the ampoule firmly, you will place your thumb on the top portion of the ampoule "the head" closest to you and quickly push your thumb forward and "snap" the head of the ampoule off. If you don't succeed your first try, score the neck again and repeat the procedure.

If your Hcg comes in a vial, you will want to snap, pry, or pop the plastic top off the vial with your finger or thumb nail.

41

Once the plastic cap is removed, you will discover an exposed circle of rubber. Later you will be sticking a needle through the rubber circle to extract your Hcg from the vial.

Now that we know how to open the ampoule/vial of Hcg, let's get started.

Step 2- Take your 10 ml/cc syringe and twist a 22, 23, or 25 gauge needle onto the tip of it.

The needle screws on clockwise. Make sure the needle is twisted/screwed all the way on the syringe. The needle should twist at least ¼ turn. If it doesn't twist at least ¼ turn, chances are that it is not screwed on and may come off during the mixing process.

Step 3 - Fill the syringe completely with distilled water.
Once the syringe is completely filled with distilled water, stand over the sink, point the needle toward the ceiling and slowly push the plunger until you have exactly 10 cc/ml of distilled water and no large air bubbles (pointed at the ceiling, the top of the black rubber plunger should be on the 10cc/ml mark)

Step 4- Once you have 10 cc/ml of distilled water in the syringe (and no large air bubbles) you will then inject the distilled water into the 30 cc/ml amber sealed vial.

Keep in mind that the vial is vacuumed sealed and when the plunger gets hard to push, you need to let go of the plunger and let it suck up air from the vial. You may need to repeat this process 2 or 3 times to get all the distilled water into the vial.

Step 5 - Once the 10 cc/ml of distilled water is in the vacuumed sealed vial, repeat the process using 3 cc/ml of flavored vodka.

Now you should have 10 cc/ml of distilled water and 3 cc/ml of flavored vodka in a 30 ml amber sealed vial.

Step 6 – Take a 3cc/ml syringe and screw a 22 or 23 guage needle on it. Fill that syringe with   two (2) cc/ml of distilled water and add it to your Hcg.

IMPORTANT: When adding the water to the Hcg, you must do it slowly so the mixture does not bubble/foam up.

When the water contacts the Hcg powder, the powder will just disappear. If the powder does not completely dissolve (disappear), then you need to gently swirl the mixture until it dissolves.

Step 7 - Once the mixture is dissolved, you need to extract it from the ampoule/vial.

You want to extract every drop possible. The 1 ½ inch needle will just reach the bottom of the ampoule/vial. If you are using a smaller or shorter needle, you may need to turn the ampoule/vial upside down and insert the needle until it just penetrates the rubber stopper, and then suck the Hcg out of the ampoule/vial (you can actually turn an open ampoule upside down and the Hcg will not flow out).

Step 8 - Take the two (2) cc/ml of mixture (Hcg and distilled water) and inject it into the amber, vacuumed-sealed vial.

Now in the amber sealed vial, you should have the following 3 liquids combined:
- 10 cc/ml of distilled water
- 3 cc/ml of clear flavored vodka
- 2 cc/ml of distilled water and Hcg mixed together
- Your amber sealed vial should be halfway full with this mixture

This will give you 15 cc/ml of liquid. You will be using ½ cc/ml 2 times a day. In total you will be using 1 cc/ml per day. Each 5000 iu bottle of Hcg will last 15 days.

Step 9 - Once the Hcg is in a vacuum sealed vial, wrap the vial in tinfoil so no light can reach the Hcg.

Step 10 - Place the tinfoil wrapped Hcg in the refrigerator.
DO NOT FREEZE THE Hcg once you have combined it into a liquid.

Once mixed into a liquid, Hcg will remain potent for 24-31 days.

Caution: Mixed Hcg left out at room temperature will lose its potency somewhere between 25-48 hours.

Now that Your Hcg is Mixed and Refrigerated, It's Time to Feast!!!

<u>A few important notes first!</u>

- Do not start the diet unless you have a complete cycle of Hcg in your possession.
- Once you reach your goal weight you are only ½ way done with the program
- **The maintenance part of the program is more important than the weight loss part of the program!**
- Plan ahead for a total of 3-12 weeks of weight loss and then 6 weeks of maintenance.
- **The biggest reason people fail on this program is that they skip out on the maintenance part of the program once they reach their desired weight.**
- It is not recommended to stay on the Very Low Calorie Diet (VLCD) for more than 12 weeks.

People who follow the program to the end, enjoy a metabolism that is restored to normal! People that don't, end up "kicking themselves" and repeating the program again at a later date.

Three (3) to twelve (12) weeks of focus and consistency = a whole new life.

"I do not know of, or have ever heard of, one person who has followed and completed this program and not achieved dramatic and noticeable weight loss" - Mark Pirkl, Author

Phase One - Loading

In the original protocol by Dr A.T.W. Simeons' and in Kevin Trudeau's book, the loading phase lasts for two (2) days. After watching my first dozen or so clients/friends suffer hunger pains their first 5-10 days of the program (because they only loaded for two (2) days), I increased the loading phase to 4-6 days. This cured the hunger pains for all future clients.

I have had several clients/friends gain up to 16 pounds during their loading phase. I was delighted when every single person lost the weight they gained within the first week of their program. I experienced an interesting observation - people who gained the most weight during their loading phase, ended up having the best overall results on the program.

The moral of the story is, "Don't be afraid to gain weight during the loading program." The more weight you gain during loading, the better results you will most likely experience overall.

As soon as you take your first dose, you can begin loading.

To take your first dose of Hcg:
- Insert the needle (that is hopefully firmly screwed on the syringe) into the vacuum sealed vial.
- Turn the vial upside down.

- When the vial is upside down and the syringe is below the vial, fill the syringe

  to the 1 cc/ml line.
- Push .5 cc/ml back into the bottle so you have .5 cc/ml mixture in the syringe and no large air bubbles.
- Holding the syringe a safe distance from your mouth (at least 1-2 inches), squirt the mixture into your mouth. If you are not comfortable doing this, take the needle cover and slide it over the needle and unscrew the needle from the syringe and then squirt the mixture into your mouth.
- Let the mixture roll under your tongue and hold it there for at least five (5) minutes before swallowing.

It is best to not eat 10 minutes before or 10 minutes after taking the mixture.

After you have taken the mixture, don't forget to wrap your vacuum sealed vial (amber colored vial) of mixture with tinfoil and immediately put it back into the fridge. You are wrapping it in tinfoil to keep any light from reaching your Hcg.

The next four days you are going to take the mixture **twice a day**, once in the morning and once in the evening. Each time you take the mixture, **you are going to take ½ (0.5) cc/ml**. You will be consuming **one (1) cc/ml *total* per day**. Your amber sealed vial contains 15 cc/ml of mixture. That is enough to last you 14 or 15 days.

Now it is time to load/feast.

Begin Loading

The amount of fat you consume during this 4-day phase is going to determine your success. People who shy away from gorging on fat during this phase have below average results.

YOU WILL BE TAKING Hcg THE ENTIRE TIME YOU ARE LOADING/GORGING.

As soon as you take your first dose of Hcg, you can began to load/gorge on fat. During this phase you want to do your best to avoid carbohydrates and starches. People who eat carbohydrates and starches during this phase often experience headaches the first few days of the diet. They also experience hunger during the first 5-10 days of the diet. AVOID CARBOHYDRATES AND STARCHES AS MUCH AS POSSIBLE! This means: no pasta, no tortillas, no bread, no sugars, no potatoes, yams, squashes, or pumpkin (NO FRENCH FRIES, NO DONUTS, NO PIZZA, NO POTATO CHIPS, NO SPAGHETTI, NO SANDWICHES, NO ICE CREAM, etc.)

Most people want an exact amount of fat or calories to consume. This varies from person to person. I recommend that you try to eat 3 times as much as you normally eat each day. Make sure that each meal is mostly fat. Try to stick to the "good fats". Good fats can be found in eggs, dairy, natural oils (coconut and olive oil are the best), meat, avocados, and nuts.
At the end of each day, you should be fully satiated and by the end of the fourth day, the thought of eating one more bite of fat should make you feel "sick to your stomach".

Once you have completed 4 days of loading, you can begin the next phase and start dropping pounds.

DO NOT EVEN THINK ABOUT STARTING THE NEXT PHASE UNLESS YOU ALREADY HAVE A HIGH QUALITY DIGITAL BATHROOM SCALE. You should be able to step on and off the scale three (3) times consecutively and get the same reading each time. The scale should also weigh/read in 0.5 pound increments or smaller. I personally recommend that you purchase the "thinner" brand scale. I have seen it available at Big Lots, 3D Bed and Bath, and Bed Bath and Beyond. I bought one just recently for $40, and it was well worth it!

Phase 2 – Very Low Calorie Diet (VLCD)

The weight loss menu is very specific. It was tested and perfected by Dr. Simeons on thousands of people. Any slight alteration can end up in a significant weight gain. I have spoken to many people who ate 2 or 3 single potato chips and gained 4-5 pounds the next day.

(*Vegetarians*, please refer to the manuscript "pounds and inches" page 64. The manuscript is located in Appendix of this book.)

Breakfast: Tea or coffee in any quantity without sugar.

Only one tablespoonful of milk allowed in 24 hours. Saccharin or Stevia may be used in any amount

Lunch: **1. One whole food supplement tablet**

2. 4 ounces of chicken breast, lean buffalo steak, lean beef (97% lean or higher), veal steak, turkey breast, White Albacore Tuna, egg whites, fresh white fish, wild Chilean Sea Bass, Flounder, Sole, Halibut lobster, crab, or shrimp. ***All visible fat must be carefully removed before cooking, and the meat must be weighed raw before cooking***. It must be boiled or grilled without additional fat.

Salmon, eel, regular tuna, herring, dried or pickled fish are not allowed.

The chicken breast/turkey breast must be removed from the bird.

3. One type of vegetable only to be chosen from the following: spinach, chard, chicory, beet-greens, green salad, tomatoes, celery, fennel, onions, red radishes, cucumbers, asparagus, cabbage. **Never eat 2 vegetables together at one meal unless one of the two vegetables is lettuce.** A tomato can be considered a fruit and can be eaten with another vegetable as long as no other fruit is eaten at that meal.

4.   An apple, a handful of strawberries or one-half grapefruit. Never eat 2 fruits at one meal.

Afternoon meal: Four (4) ounces of protein

Dinner :   The same choices as lunch

Each day you will need to drink one gallon of water or recommended liquids throughout the day. You will also need to take three 99/mg potassium tablets everyday if you are not consuming apple cider vinegar everyday!

Drinks and Seasonings

- The juice of **one** lemon daily is allowed for all purposes.

- <u>**Your body will crave sea salt and will need salt!!! Feel free to use as much of the recommended types of salt as it takes to satisfy your cravings**</u>. We are not trying to lose water weight and increased recommended salt type salt consumption will not affect your losses.   The salt must be one of the following three: Sea Salt, Himalayan Salt, Celtic Salt.

- Pepper, Apple cider vinegar, Braggs Liquid Aminos, Liquid Stevia, mustard powder, chili powder, garlic, sweet basil, parsley, thyme, majoram, red tabasco sauce, mustard, etc., may be used for seasoning, **but no oil, butter, or dressing**. (If you use red tabasco sauce or a wing type sauce make sure it is sugar, carbohydrate and calorie free.)

- Balsamic and/or red wine vinegar are <u>not</u> allowed.

- Tea, coffee, plain water, or bottled water (**1 gallon of water/liquid per day is recommended**) are the only drinks allowed, but they may be taken in any quantity and at all times.

It's pretty simple; if it isn't on the menu, don't eat it.

Don't try to improvise. Don't try to substitute for foods that aren't on the menu. If you follow the program exactly, you will have unbelievable success.

You will be consuming 500 calories a day, and the Hcg is going to allow your body to release your abnormal fat stores to satisfy your body's daily caloric need. In other words, if my body needs 2600 calories a day, I will be eating 500 calories and my body will be releasing 2100 calories of abnormally stored fat to compensate for the difference.

Eating less than 500 calories a day can often slow down or stop the body from releasing the stored fat. Every day you want to make sure you come as close as you can to your 500 calorie recommended daily intake! Each day it is MANDATORY that you eat 8-12 ounces of protein.

Try to keep in mind while on phase two (VLCD) the lower you keep your carbohydrate and fat intake, the faster you will lose weight. I have designed the following two charts to help you figure out how much carbohydrates, calories and fats are in the foods on the VLCD menu. The following information was taken from www.calorieking.com.

NUTRITIONAL CONTENT OF PROTEIN
www.calorieking.com

PROTEIN	Qty	cal	fat (g)	Sat. fat (g)	chol (mg)	protein
96% lean ground beef pan fried	4 oz	185	6.7	3	86	29.2
veal steak sirloin roasted	4 oz	190	7	2.7	118	29.7
chicken breast skinless	4 oz	120	1.6	0.4	64	26.4
wild Chilean sea bass	4 oz	112	2.4	0.4	48	20.8
Flounder	4 oz	104	1.2	0.4	64	21.6
Sole	4 oz	104	1.2	0.4	64	21.6
Halibut	4 oz	124	2.8	0.4	36	23.6
fresh white fish	4 oz	104	1.6	0.4	76	20.8

lobster with-out the shell cooked	4 oz	106	2.8	1.5	70	18.2
crab no shell baked broiled	4 oz	40.7	1.9	0.33	28	5.62
buffalo steak	4 oz	125	2.13	0.8	72	25
shrimp	4 oz	120	2	0.4	173	23.1
turkey breast	4 oz	118	1.9	0.5	49	19.4
ostrich	4 oz	114	2	0	45	24
albacore tuna	4 oz	140	2	0	50	30

NUTRITIONAL CONTENT OF HCG DIET FRUITS AND VEGETABLES

www.calorieking.com

Vegetable	Qty	net carb	cal	total carb
Lettuce, Boston and Bibb butterhead	1 oz	0.3	4	0.6
Lettuce, Romaine or cos	1 oz	0.3	5	0.9
Asparagus, c, b ,d, no salt	1 oz	0.5	6	1.1
Spinach, c, b, d, no salt	1 oz	0.4	7	1
Beet Greens,c, b, d no salt	1 oz	0.1	6	1.2
Lettuce, Iceberg	1 oz	0.5	4	0.6
Cucumber, peeled, raw, diced	1 oz	0.4	3	0.6
Chard, swiss, c, b, d no salt	1 oz	0.6	5	1.1
Cabbage, c, b, d no salt	1 oz	0.9	7	1.6
Green onions, raw 8 stalks	1 oz	1.4	9	2.1
Radishes, raw	1 oz	0.5	5	1
Celery, c, b, d no salt	1 oz	0.3	4	0.8
Tomatoes, red ripe raw	1 oz	0.8	5	1.1
Fennel, bulb raw, sliced	1 oz	1.2	9	2.1

Fruits
Strawberries, halves	1 oz	1.6	9	2.2
Grapefruit, raw, pink/red all areas	1 oz	2	9	2.3
Apple, raw sliced	1 oz	3.2	15	3.9

The following *Fluctuations in weight loss, Interruptions of Weight Loss, The Plateau, and Reaching a Former Level* are taken directly from Dr. Simeon's manuscript "pounds and Inches" that is located in the appendix of this book.

Fluctuations in weight loss

After the fourth or fifth day of dieting, the daily loss of weight begins to decrease to one pound or somewhat less per day, and there is a smaller urinary output. Men often continue to lose regularly at that rate, but women are more irregular in spite of faultless dieting. There may be no drop at all for two or three days and then a sudden loss which reestablishes the normal average. These fluctuations are entirely due to variations in the retention and elimination of water, which are more marked in women than in men.

The weight registered by the scale is determined by two processes not necessarily synchronized. Under the influence of HCG, fat is being extracted from the cells, in which it is stored in the fatty tissue. When these cells are empty and therefore serve no purpose, the body breaks down the cellular structure and absorbs it, but breaking up of useless cells, connective tissue, blood vessels, etc., may lag behind the process of fat-extraction. When this happens the body appears to replace some of the extracted fat with water which is retained for this purpose. As water is heavier than fat the scales may show no loss of weight, although sufficient fat has actually been consumed to make up for the deficit in the 500-Calorie diet. When then such tissue is finally broken down, the water is liberated and there is a sudden flood of urine and a marked loss of weight. This simple interpretation of what is really an extremely complex mechanism is the one we give those patients who want to know why it is that on certain days they do not lose, though they have committed no dietary error.

Patients who have previously regularly used diuretics as a method of reducing, lose fat during the first two or three weeks of treatment which shows in their measurements, but the scale may show little or no loss because they are replacing the normal water content of their body which has been dehydrated. Diuretics should never be used for reducing.

Interruptions of Weight Loss

We distinguish four types of interruption in the regular daily loss. The first is the one that has already been mentioned in which the weight stays stationary for a day or two, and this occurs, particularly towards the end of a course, in almost every case.

The Plateau

The second type of interruption we call a "plateau". A plateau lasts 4-6 days and frequently occurs during the second half of a full course, particularly in patients that have been doing well and whose overall average of nearly a pound per effective injection has been maintained. Those who are losing more than the average all have a plateau sooner or later. A plateau always corrects, itself, but many patients who have become accustomed to a regular daily loss get unnecessarily worried and begin to fret. No amount of explanation convinces them that a plateau does not mean that they are no longer responding normally to treatment.

In such cases we consider it permissible, for purely psychological reasons, to break up the plateau. This can be done in two ways. One is a so-called "apple day". An apple-day begins at lunch and continues until just before lunch of the following day. The patients are given six large apples and are told to eat one whenever they feel the desire though six apples is the maximum allowed. During an apple-day no other food or liquids except plain water are allowed and of water they may only drink just enough to quench an uncomfortable thirst if eating an apple still leaves them thirsty. Most patients feel no need for water and are quite happy with their six apples. Needless to say, an apple-day may never be given on the day on which there is no injection. The apple-day produces a gratifying loss of weight on the following

day, chiefly due to the elimination of water. This water is not regained when the patients resume their normal 500-Calorie diet at lunch, and on the following days they continue to lose weight satisfactorily.

The other way to break up a plateau is by giving a non-mercurial diuretic[1] for one day. This is simpler for the patient but we prefer the apple-day as we sometimes find that though the diuretic is very effective on the following day it may take two to three days before the normal daily reduction is resumed, throwing the patient into a new fit of despair. It is useless to give either an apple-day or a diuretic unless the weight has been stationary for at least four days without any dietary error having been committed.

Reaching a Former Level

The third type of interruption in the regular loss of weight may last much longer - ten days to two weeks. Fortunately, it is rare and only occurs in very advanced cases, and then hardly ever during the first course of treatment. It is seen only in those patients who during some period of their lives have maintained a certain fixed degree of obesity for ten years or more and have then at some time rapidly increased beyond that weight. When then in the course of treatment the former level is reached, it may take two weeks of no loss, in spite of HCG and diet, before further reduction is normally resumed.

Important Highlights for Phase 2 – The VLCD:

- ***You should continue ALL doctor prescribed medications until the doctor instructs you otherwise.***

- No nonprescription medicines or cosmetics other than lipstick, eyebrow pencil, and powder should be used.

- Individuals that weigh themselves every morning (after going to the bathroom and before eating their first meal of the day) and write their daily food intake down, **always** report better results than individuals that don't weigh and record their results.   (Important: **a great website** to calculate your caloric intake and record your daily weight and progress is: **www.fitday.com)**

- Mild headaches are common the first 3 days. This is due to carbohydrate withdrawal. Only aspirin is approved as a pain reliever.

- Constipation is common. It can be cured with smooth move tea, oxygenated magnesium, or an Enema. Many past dieters took 1-3 capsules of oxygenated magnesium a day with great success.

- **Some people experience` cramping**. This can be cured by taking **three 99mg potassium tablets a day**. Potassium tablets are cheap and can be found at any store in the women's vitamin section. Apple Cider Vinegar is also high in potassium. Dieters who consume Apple Cider Vinegar every day, on salads or on cucumber slices, never seem to experience muscle cramping.

- If your skin is dry and flaky, you need to increase your water/fluid intake.

- **The most effective plan is to eat 3 meals a day** and to make **sure that you eat 4 ounces of protein at each meal.** *A big first meal of the day seems to stave off any hunger for the day.*

- I recommend a big salad with chopped meat in it for the first meal (brunch/lunch) using a combination of Apple Cider Vinegar, Water, Liquid Stevia & Braggs liquid Aminos as seasoning. Three (3) meals of 4-ounces of protein will be between 300-360 calories and then you can split the remaining calories up between vegetables and fruit.

- Strawberries, cabbage, onions, and sometimes tomatoes have been reported to slow down weight loss for a certain percentage of people.

- People that consume no fruit and eat only meat and vegetables, seem to get the best results.

- Cucumber slices in a combination of Braggs Apple Cider Vinegar, Braggs Liquid Aminos, and Stevia make a great snack to snack on throughout the day.

- You will be on the edge of protein deficiency, and you ***must always consume at least 8 ounces of meat/fish/protein a day.***

- Latex gloves should be worn when trimming the excess fat off of meat.

- If you are weak or tired during the day, **it is *almost always due to not eating enough protein***

- Meals can be broken up and eaten at different times.

- Some people can drink diet soda, and it doesn't affect their weight loss. This is a personal choice, and **no diet soda should be consumed until you have lost at least 10 pounds** and can see the effect of having a diet drink on your weight loss program.

- The 500-600 calorie limit must always be maintained.

- 2 small apples are not an acceptable exchange for "1 large apple."

- 4 ounces of non-fat Cottage cheese made from skimmed milk may occasionally be substituted for meat/fish.

- Lean ground beef has to be 96% (or higher) lean.

Personal Care and Beauty Products on the Hcg Diet:

- We do permit the use of lipstick, powder and such lotions as are entirely free of fatty substances. We also allow brilliantine to be used on the hair but it must not be rubbed into the scalp. Obviously sun-tan oil is prohibited.

- Aspirin and birth control **are** allowed on the Hcg Diet.

- No oil type massage of any kind is allowed. Thermal massage beds (Migun) are ok to use.

- A short list of Hcg Diet-friendly personal care and beauty products are available here: http://www.hcgdietinfo.com/HCG-Diet-Products.htm

For those of you worried about the 500 calorie a day restriction, please read the following paragraph that is taken directly from Dr Simeon's manuscript "pounds and inches" located in the back of this book:

> "Just as the daily dose of HCG is the same in all cases, so the same diet proves to be satisfactory for a small elderly lady of leisure or a hard working muscular giant. Under the effect of HCG the obese body is always able to obtain all the Calories it needs from the abnormal fat deposits, regardless of whether it uses up 1500 or 4000 per day. It must be made very clear to the patient that he is living to a far greater extent on the fat which he is losing than on what he eats."

Getting Bored of Eating the Same Thing?

A former Hcg dieter and chef has written a cookbook for Hcg dieters that is worth its weight in gold. I don't know her, nor do I have any financial interest in referring people to her. When I first did the Hcg diet, I didn't know about her cookbook. Since then, I have had several friends purchase the cookbook and rave about it. She has included gourmet recipes that most people can use for the rest of their lives.

For more information on this remarkable cookbook you can go to: http://www.hcgrecipes.com.

Reaching Your Goal Weight

Once you have completed at least 23 days of the (VLCD) diet **and** you are at your goal, you can start the next phase, Phase 3 (maintenance).

It takes 23 days on the VLCD to reset your metabolism. **If you reached your goal before completing 23 days of the VLCD, do the following;**

- Continue to eat exactly the same menu that you have been eating

- Increase your daily calories to maintain your weight

- Continue on the increased calories and VLCD menu until you have completed a full 23 days of the VLCD menu

IMPORTANT: Before you start Phase 3, you need to make sure you record the weight you were at when you took your last dose of Hcg (**last dosing weight = LDW**).

Your Last Dosing Weight (LDW) is what you weighed the day you took your last/final dose of Hcg. **YOUR LDW NUMBER IS VERY IMPORTANT!**

Phase 3 – Stabilizing Your Metabolism and Setting Your Body's Weight Set Point

This phase is the most important phase!!! This is the phase that is going to set your body's metabolism to your body's new weight.

Dieters who complete this phase correctly enjoy a restored metabolism!!! Dieters who skip this phase will most likely regain some or all of the weight they lost!

Phase 3 Overview

- Write down your current weight (LDW)

- Stop taking Hcg and stay on current diet and calories for 3 more days (72 more hours) while Hcg leaves your system

- On day 4 increase your calories to a "normal" recommended calorie level

- Slowly add fats to your VLCD diet while maintaining your weight within 2 pounds of your last dosing weight. This continues for 3 weeks

- Once you reach 3 weeks, slowly start adding carbohydrates and starches to your current diet

- Continue adding carbohydrates and starches for the next 3 weeks while staying within 2 pounds of your last dosing weight

- Once the 6 weeks is over (3 weeks of adding fats and 3 more of adding fats and carbs), your metabolism should be stabilized and adjusted to your current calorie intake. Your metabolism should also be adjusted to a "normal" carbohydrate and fat intake.

Beginning Phase 3

For the first three (3) days of Phase 3, you are going to continue eating exactly the same. The same amount of calories and the same VLCD menu you have been eating (for most Hcg dieters, this will be 500 calories a day).

You are going to stop taking the Hcg immediately!

You will stay on the same calories/menu (500 calories for most Hcg'ers) for the next three days (72 hours after taking your last dose of Hcg) while the Hcg leaves your system.

Once 72 hours have passed with-out taking Hcg you can increase your calories.

You now need to increase your calories to maintain your current weight.

You need to figure out how many calories you need to eat to stay at your current weight.

Author's note: Many websites I have researched recommend taking your current bodyweight and multiplying it by 12 for men and by 11 for women. This is a basic calculation. **It is a starting point!** It may need to be adjusted by you due to your metabolic rate and level of exercise (This calculation may be too high or too low for some individuals, due to how many calories their body is burning off each day).

MEN:

For example, a **male** that now weighs 203 pounds would calculate **his** daily recommended calorie intake by taking **his** weight, 203, and multiplying it by 12.

203 x 12 = 2436 calories a day

That **male** would immediately increase **his** caloric intake to 2436 a day.

WOMEN:

For example, a **female** that now weighs 134 pounds would calculate **her** daily recommended calorie intake by taking **her** current weight, 134 and multiplying it by 11.

134 x 11 = 1474 calories a day

This **female** would immediately increase **her** caloric intake to 1474 calories a day.

For the next 6 weeks, your weight needs to stay within (+) or (-) two pounds of your last dosing weight (the weight you were at on your last dose of Hcg).

It may take your body a few days to get used to the increased calorie intake. Many people can't consume the new calorie intake due to the fact that they "feel too full" before they reach their recommended daily calorie intake.

I recommend not adding any new fats to your VLCD diet for 2 or 3 days while you adjust to the increased calorie intake.

For the next 21 days you will slowly add fats to your diet. Healthy fats are the most recommended. Some healthy fats are coconut oil, (one of the healthiest fats you can consume) olive oil, most oil made from nuts, cheese, meat, avocados, dairy products (yogurt, cottage cheese, butter, etc.) peanut butter, nut butter, etc.

Ex; one day have eggs with cheese and food from the VLCD menu. See how your body reacts as far as weight gain or loss is concerned. The next day have some kind of meat and food from the VLCD menu. The following day snack on some nuts during the day and eat food from the VLCD menu. The next day have some peanut butter and food from the VLCD menu. Keep adding fats slowly each day to your diet.

A product that is Hcg Diet friendly and that many Hcg'ers really like is called Carbmaster Yogurt and it can be currently purchased at Kroger grocery stores in the USA.

During this time you need to remember to stay within plus or minus 2 pounds of your LDW.

If you drop below 2 pounds of your LDW, all you need to do is increase your caloric intake immediately! If you go above 2 pounds of your LDW, then you need to do what is called a "Skipping a Meal/Steak Day."

The following (**"skipping a meal"**, **"losing more weight"**) is taken from Dr. Simeons manuscript "pounds and inches" located in the back of this book:

"Skipping a Meal"

As long as their weight stays within two pounds of the weight reached on the day of the last injection, patients should take no notice of any increase but the moment the scale goes beyond two pounds, even if this is only a few ounces, they must on that same day entirely skip breakfast and lunch but take plenty to drink. In the evening they must eat a huge steak with only an apple or a raw tomato. Of course this rule applies only to the morning weight. Ex-obese patients should never check their weight during the day, as there may be wide fluctuations and these are merely alarming and confusing. It is of utmost importance that the meal is skipped on the same day as the scale registers an increase of more than two pounds and that missing the meals is not postponed until the following day. If a meal is skipped on the day in which a gain is registered in the morning this brings about an immediate drop of often over a pound. But if the skipping of the meal - and skipping means literally skipping, not just having a light meal - is postponed the phenomenon does not occur and several days of strict dieting may be necessary to correct the situation.

Most patients hardly ever need to skip a meal. If they have eaten a heavy lunch they feel no desire to eat their dinner, and in this case no increase takes place. If they keep their weight at the point reached at the end of the treatment, even a heavy dinner does not bring about an increase of two pounds on the next morning and does not therefore call for any special measures. Most patients are surprised how small their appetite has become and yet how much they can eat without gaining weight. They no longer suffer from an abnormal appetite and feel satisfied with much less food than before. In fact, they are usually disappointed that they cannot manage their first normal meal, which they have been planning for weeks.

"Losing more Weight"

An ex-patient should never gain more than two pounds without immediately correcting this, but it is equally undesirable that more than two lbs. be lost after treatment, because a greater loss is always achieved at the expense of normal fat. Any normal fat that is lost is invariably regained as soon as more food is taken, and it often happens that this rebound overshoots the upper two lbs. limit."

Once you have completed 21 days of adding fats to your VLCD diet, you are slowly going to start adding carbohydrates and starches to your diet. You will slowly add them just as you did with the fats.

For the next 21 days you are going to slowly add carbohydrates, sugars and starches to your VLCD diet that now includes fats.

 Starches should be added last.

Dangerous starches (starches that make most people gain weight easily include; POTATOES, SQUASH, PUMPKIN, BEANS, WHEAT, YAMS, SWEET POTATOES). Potatoes seem to be the worst offender when it comes to weight gain.

Very sweet fruits, pastries and sugary foods can also cause fast weight gain!

The following is taken from Dr Simeon's manuscript "pounds and inches:"

It takes about 3 weeks before the weight reached at the end of the treatment becomes stable, i.e. does not show violent fluctuations after an occasional excess. During this period, patients must realize that the so-called carbohydrates, that is sugar, rice, bread, potatoes, pastries, etc, are by far the most dangerous. If no carbohydrates whatsoever are eaten, fats can be indulged in somewhat more liberally and even small quantities of alcohol, such as a glass of wine with meals, does no harm, but **as soon as fats and starch are combined things are very liable to get out of hand.** This has to be observed very carefully during the first 3 weeks after the treatment is ended otherwise disappointments are almost sure to occur.

Congratulations!

Once you have completed the six weeks of adding fats, carbohydrates, starches, and sugars to your diet and have stayed within 2 pounds of your LDW, you have completed the program. You should enjoy a metabolism that is "restored to normal."

To maintain your healthy new lifestyle, moderate exercise (cardiovascular and weight training) is highly recommended.

Relapses

The following is an excerpt from Dr. Simeon's manuscript called "Pounds and Inches:"

Relapses

As a general rule one can say that 60%-70% of our cases experience little or no difficulty in holding their weight permanently. Relapses may be due to negligence in the basic rule of daily weighing. Many patients think that this is unnecessary and that they can judge any increase from the fit of their clothes. Some do not carry their scale with them on a journey as it is cumbersome and takes a big bite out of their luggage-allowance when flying. This is a disastrous mistake, because after a course of HCG as much as 10 lbs. can be regained without any noticeable change in the fit of the clothes. The reason for this is that after treatment newly acquired fat is at first evenly distributed and does not show the former preference for certain parts of the body.

Pregnancy or the menopause may annul the effect of a previous treatment. Women who take treatment during the one year after the last menstruation - that is at the onset of the menopause - do just as well as others, but among them the relapse rate is higher until the menopause is fully established. The period of one year after the last menstruation applies only to women who are not being treated with ovarian hormones. If these are taken, the premenopausal period may be indefinitely prolonged.

Late teenage girls who suffer from attacks of compulsive eating have by far the worst record of all as far as relapses are concerned.

Patients who have once taken the treatment never seem to hesitate to come back for another short course as soon as they notice that their weight is once again getting out of hand. They come quite cheerfully and hopefully, assured that they can be helped again. Repeat courses are often even more satisfactory than the first treatment and have the advantage, as do second courses that the patient already, knows that he will feel comfortable throughout.

Losing More Weight - Additional Courses

The following is an excerpt from Dr Simeon's "Pounds and Inches" manuscript:

Further Courses

Patients requiring the loss of more than 34 lbs. must have a second or even more courses. A second course can be started after an interval of not less than six weeks, though the pause can be more than six weeks. When a third, fourth or even fifth course is necessary, the interval between courses should be made

progressively longer. Between a second and third course eight weeks should elapse, between a third and fourth course twelve weeks, between a fourth and fifth course twenty weeks and between a fifth and sixth course six months. In this way it is possible to bring about a weight reduction of 100 lbs. and more if required without the least hardship to the patient.

In general, men do slightly better than women and often reach a somewhat higher average daily loss. Very advanced cases do a little better than early ones, but it is a remarkable fact that this difference is only just statistically significant.

A Final Note from the Author

I truly hope that this book will change your life. I appreciate you spending your hard earned money on it.

I am currently researching some natural appetite suppressants that look promising. When I find an affordable and healthy product, I will try my best to relay the information to all my readers.

If you would like to hire a personal guide to maximize your results, please contact me at markpirkl@ymail.com. All guides are former Hcg weight loss clients who have first -hand experience with this program. Dieters who have hired these personal guides in the past have all achieved "above average" results on their Hcg weight loss program.

Best wishes on your new life,

Mark Pirkl

Appendix

POUNDS AND INCHES

A New Approach to Obesity

BY

A.T.W. SIMEONS M.D.

SALVATOR MUNDI INTERNATIONAL HOSPITAL

00152 - ROME

VIALE MURA GIANICOLENSI, 77

SEVENTH EDITION

1971

FOREWORD

This book discusses a new interpretation of the nature of obesity, and while it does not advocate yet another fancy slimming diet it does describe a method of treatment which has grown out of theoretical considerations based on clinical observation.

What I have to say is an essence of views distilled out of forty years of grappling with the fundamental problems of obesity, its causes, its symptoms, and its very nature. In these many years of specialized work, thousands of cases have passed through my hands and were carefully studied. Every new theory, every new method, every promising lead was considered, experimentally screened and critically evaluated as soon as it became known. But invariably the results were disappointing and lacking in uniformity.

I felt that we were merely nibbling at the fringe of a great problem, as, indeed, do most serious students of overweight. We have grown pretty sure that the tendency to accumulate abnormal fat is a very definite metabolic disorder, much as is, for instance, diabetes. Yet the localization and the nature of this disorder remained a mystery. Every new approach seemed to lead into a blind alley, and though patients were told that they are fat because they eat too much, we believed that this is neither the whole truth nor the last word in the matter.

Refusing to be side-tracked by an all too facile interpretation of obesity, I have always held that overeating is the result of the disorder, not its cause, and that we can make little headway until we can build for ourselves some sort of theoretical structure with which to explain the condition. Whether such a structure represents the truth is not important at this moment. What it must do is to give us an intellectually satisfying interpretation of what is happening in the obese body. It must also be able to withstand the onslaught of all hitherto known clinical facts and furnish a hard background against which the results of treatment can be accurately assessed.

To me this requirement seems basic, and it has always been the center of my interest. In dealing with obese patients it became a habit to register and order every clinical experience as if it were an odd looking piece of a jig-saw puzzle. And then, as in a jig saw puzzle, little clusters of fragments began to form, though they seemed to fit in nowhere. As the years passed these clusters grew bigger and started to amalgamate until, about sixteen years ago, a complete picture became dimly discernible. This picture was, and still is, dotted with gaps for which I cannot find the pieces, but I do now feel that a theoretical structure is visible as a whole.

With mounting experience, more and more facts seemed to fit snugly into the new framework, and when then a treatment based on such speculations showed consistently satisfactory results, I was sure that some practical advance had been made, regardless of whether the theoretical interpretation of these results is correct or not.

The clinical results of the new treatment have been published in scientific journal[2] and these reports have been generally well received by the profession, but the very nature of a scientific article does not permit the full presentation of new theoretical concepts nor is there room to discuss the finer points of technique and the reasons for observing them.

During the 16 years that have elapsed since I first published my findings, I have had many hundreds of inquiries from research institutes, doctors and patients. Hitherto I could only refer those interested to my scientific papers, though I realized that these did not contain sufficient information to enable doctors to conduct the new treatment satisfactorily. Those who tried were obliged to gain their own experience through the many trials and errors which I have long since overcome.

Doctors from all over the world have come to Italy to study the method, first hand in my clinic in the Salvator Mundi International Hospital in Rome. For some of them the time they could spare has been too short to get a full grasp of the technique, and in any case the number of those whom I have been able to meet personally is small compared with the many requests for further detailed information which keep coming in. I have tried to keep up with these demands by correspondence, but the volume of this work has become unmanageable and that is one excuse for writing this book.

In dealing with a disorder in which the patient must take an active part in the treatment, it is, I believe, essential that he or she have an understanding of what is being done and why. Only then can there be intelligent cooperation between physician and patient. In order to avoid writing two books, one for the physician and another for the patient - a prospect which would probably have resulted in no book at all - I have tried to meet the requirements of both in a single book. This is a rather difficult enterprise in which I may not have succeeded. The expert will grumble about long-windedness while the lay-reader may occasionally have to look up an unfamiliar word in the glossary provided for him.

---

[2] A list of references to the more important articles is given at the end of this booklet.

To make the text more readable I shall be unashamedly authoritative and avoid all the hedging and tentativeness with which it is customary to express new scientific concepts grown out of clinical experience and not as yet confirmed by clear-cut laboratory experiments. Thus, when I make what reads like a factual statement, the professional reader may have to translate into: clinical experience seems to suggest that such and such an observation might be tentatively explained by such and such a working hypothesis, requiring a vast amount of further research before the hypothesis can be considered a valid theory. If we can from the outset establish this as a mutually accepted convention, I hope to avoid being accused of speculative exuberance.

Obesity a Disorder

As a basis for our discussion we postulate that obesity in all its many forms is due to an abnormal functioning of some part of the body and that every ounce of abnormally accumulated fat is always the result of the same disorder of certain regulatory mechanisms. Persons suffering from this particular disorder will get fat regardless of whether they eat excessively, normally or less than normal. A person who is free of the disorder will never get fat, even if he frequently overeats.

Those in whom the disorder is severe will accumulate fat very rapidly, those in whom it is moderate will gradually increase in weight and those in whom it is mild may be able to keep their excess weight stationary for long periods. In all these cases a loss of weight brought about by dieting, treatments with thyroid, appetite-reducing drugs, laxatives, violent exercise, massage, baths, etc., is only temporary and will be rapidly regained as soon as the reducing regimen is relaxed. The reason is simply that none of these measures corrects the basic disorder.

While there are great variations in the severity of obesity, we shall consider all the different forms in both sexes and at all ages as always being due to the same disorder. Variations in form would then be partly a matter of degree, partly an inherited bodily constitution and partly the result of a secondary involvement of endocrine glands such as the pituitary, the thyroid, the adrenals or the sex glands. On the other hand, we postulate that no deficiency of any of these glands can ever directly produce the common disorder known as obesity.

If this reasoning is correct, it follows that a treatment aimed at curing the disorder must be equally effective in both sexes, at all ages and in all forms of obesity. Unless this is so, we are entitled to harbor grave doubts as to whether a given treatment corrects the underlying disorder. Moreover, any claim that the disorder has been corrected must be substantiated by the ability of the patient to eat normally of any food he pleases without regaining abnormal fat after treatment. Only if these conditions are fulfilled can we legitimately speak of curing obesity rather than of reducing weight.

Our problem thus presents itself as an enquiry into the localization and the nature of the disorder which leads to obesity. The history of this enquiry is a long series of high hopes and bitter disappointments.

The History of Obesity

There was a time, not so long ago, when obesity was considered a sign of health and prosperity in man and of beauty, amorousness and fecundity in women. This attitude probably dates back to Neolithic times, about 8000 years ago; when for the first time in the history of culture, man began to own property, domestic animals, arable land, houses, pottery and metal tools. Before that, with the possible exception of some races such as the Hottentots, obesity was almost non-existent, as it still is in all wild animals and most primitive races.

Today obesity is extremely common among all civilized races, because a disposition to the disorder can be inherited. Wherever abnormal fat was regarded as an asset, sexual selection tended to propagate the trait. It is only in very recent times that manifest obesity has lost some of its allure, though the cult of the outsize bust - always a sign of latent obesity - shows that the trend still lingers on.

The Significance of Regular Meals

In the early Neolithic times another change took place which may well account for the fact that today nearly all inherited dispositions sooner or later develop into manifest obesity. This change was the institution of regular meals. In pre-Neolithic times, man ate only when he was hungry and only as much as he required to still the pangs of hunger. Moreover, much of his food was raw and all of it was unrefined. He roasted his meat, but he did not boil it, as he had no pots, and what little he may have grubbed from the Earth and picked from the trees, he ate as he went along.

The whole structure of man's omnivorous digestive tract is, like that of an ape, rat or pig, adjusted to the continual nibbling of tidbits. It is not suited to occasional gorging as is, for instance, the intestine of the carnivorous cat family. Thus the institution of regular meals, particularly of food rendered rapidly assimilable, placed a great burden on modern man's ability to cope with large quantities of food suddenly pouring into his system from the intestinal tract.

The institution of regular meals meant that man had to eat more than his body required at the moment of eating so as to tide him over until the next meal. Food rendered easily digestible suddenly flooded his body with nourishment of which he was in no need at the moment. Somehow, somewhere this surplus had to be stored.

Three Kinds of Fat

In the human body we can distinguish three kinds of fat. The first is the structural fat which fills the gaps between various organs, a sort of packing material. Structural fat also performs such important functions as bedding the kidneys in soft elastic tissue, protecting the coronary arteries and keeping the skin smooth and taut. It also provides the springy cushion of hard fat under the bones of the feet, without which we would be unable to walk.

The second type of fat is a normal reserve of fuel upon which the body can freely draw when the nutritional income from the intestinal tract is insufficient to meet the demand. Such normal reserves are localized all over the body. Fat is a substance which packs the highest caloric value into the smallest space so that normal reserves of fuel for muscular activity and the maintenance of body temperature can be most economically stored in this form. Both these types of fat, structural and reserve, are normal, and even if the body stocks them to capacity this can never be called obesity.

But there is a third type of fat which is entirely abnormal. It is the accumulation of such fat, and of such fat only, from which the overweight patient suffers. This abnormal fat is also a potential reserve of fuel, but unlike the normal reserves it is not available to the body in a nutritional emergency. It is, so to speak, locked away in a fixed deposit and is not kept in a current account[3], as are the normal reserves.

When an obese patient tries to reduce by starving himself, he will first lose his normal fat reserves. When these are exhausted he begins to burn up structural fat, and only as a last resort will the body yield its abnormal reserves, though by that time the patient usually feels so weak and hungry that the diet is abandoned. It is just for this reason that obese patients complain that when they diet they lose the wrong fat. They feel famished and tired and their face becomes drawn and haggard, but their belly, hips, thighs and upper arms show little improvement. The fat they have come to detest stays on and the fat they need to cover their bones gets less and less. Their skin wrinkles and they look old and miserable. And that is one of the most frustrating and depressing experiences a human being can have.

Injustice to the Obese

When then obese patients are accused of cheating, gluttony, lack of will power, greed and sexual complexes, the strong become indignant and decide that modern medicine is a fraud and its representatives fools, while the weak just give up the struggle in despair. In either case the result is the same: a further gain in weight, resignation to an abominable fate and the resolution at least to live tolerably the short span allotted to them - a fig for doctors and insurance companies.

Obese patients only feel physically well as long as they are stationary or gaining weight. They may feel guilty, owing to the lethargy and indolence always associated with obesity. They may feel ashamed of what they have been led to believe is a lack of control. They may feel horrified by the appearance of their nude body and the tightness of

---

[3] "Current account" is the British name for what Americans call a checking account.

their clothes. But they have a primitive feeling of animal content which turns to misery and suffering as soon as they make a resolute attempt to reduce. For this there are sound reasons.

In the first place, more caloric energy is required to keep a large body at a certain temperature than to heat a small body. Secondly the muscular effort of moving a heavy body is greater than in the case of a light body. The muscular effort consumes Calories which must be provided by food. Thus, all other factors being equal, a fat person requires more food than a lean one. One might therefore reason that if a fat person eats only the additional food his body requires he should be able to keep his weight stationary. Yet every physician who has studied obese patients under rigorously controlled conditions knows that this is not true.

Many obese patients actually gain weight on a diet which is calorically deficient for their basic needs. There must thus be some other mechanism at work.

Glandular Theories

At one time it was thought that this mechanism might be concerned with the sex glands. Such a connection was suggested by the fact that many juvenile obese patients show an under-development of the sex organs. The middle-age spread in men and the tendency of many women to put on weight in the menopause seemed to indicate a causal connection between diminishing sex function and overweight. Yet, when highly active sex hormones became available, it was found that their administration had no effect whatsoever on obesity. The sex glands could therefore not be the seat of the disorder.

The Thyroid Gland

When it was discovered that the thyroid gland controls the rate at which body-fuel is consumed, it was thought that by administering thyroid gland to obese patients their abnormal fat deposits could be burned up more rapidly. This too proved to be entirely disappointing, because as we now know, these abnormal deposits take no part in the body's energy-turnover - they are inaccessibly locked away. Thyroid medication merely forces the body to consume its normal fat reserves, which are already depleted in obese patients, and then to break down structurally essential fat without touching the abnormal deposits. In this way a patient may be brought to the brink of starvation in spite of having a hundred pounds of fat to spare. Thus any weight loss brought about by thyroid medication is always at the expense of fat of which the body is in dire need.

While the majority of obese patients have a perfectly normal thyroid gland and some even have an overactive thyroid, one also occasionally sees a case with a real thyroid deficiency. In such cases, treatment with thyroid brings about a small loss of weight, but this is not due to the loss of any abnormal fat. It is entirely the result of the elimination of a mucoid substance, called myxedema, which the body accumulates when there is a marked primary thyroid deficiency. Moreover, patients suffering only from a severe lack of thyroid hormone never become obese in the true sense. Possibly also the observation that normal persons - though not the obese - lose weight rapidly when their thyroid becomes overactive may have contributed to the false notion that thyroid deficiency and obesity are connected. Much misunderstanding about the supposed role of the thyroid gland in obesity is still met with, and it is now really high time that thyroid preparations be once and for all struck off the list of remedies for obesity. This is particularly so because giving thyroid gland to an obese patient whose thyroid is either normal or overactive, besides being useless, is decidedly dangerous.

The Pituitary Gland

The next gland to be falsely incriminated was the anterior lobe of the pituitary, or hypophysis. This most important gland lies well protected in a bony capsule at the base of the skull. It has a vast number of functions in the body, among which is the regulation of all the other important endocrine glands. The fact that various signs of anterior pituitary deficiency are often associated with obesity raised the hope that the seat of the disorder might be in this gland. But although a large number of pituitary hormones have been isolated and many extracts of the gland prepared, not a single one or any combination of such factors proved to be of any value in the treatment of obesity. Quite recently, however, a fat-mobilizing factor has been found in pituitary glands, but it is still too early to say whether this factor is destined to play a role in the treatment of obesity.

The Adrenals

Recently, a long series of brilliant discoveries concerning the working of the adrenal or suprarenal glands, small bodies which sit atop the kidneys, have created tremendous interest. This interest also turned to the problem of obesity when it was discovered that a condition which in some respects resembles a severe case of obesity - the so called Cushing's Syndrome - was caused by a glandular new-growth of the adrenals or by their excessive stimulation with ACTH, which is the pituitary hormone governing the activity of the outer rind or cortex of the adrenals.

When we learned that an abnormal stimulation of the adrenal cortex could produce signs that resemble true obesity, this knowledge furnished no practical means of treating obesity by decreasing the activity of the adrenal cortex. There is no evidence to suggest that in obesity there is any excess of adrenocortical activity; in fact, all the evidence points to the contrary. There seems to be rather a lack of adrenocortical function and a decrease in the secretion of ACTH from the anterior pituitary lobe.[4]

So here again our search for the mechanism which produces obesity led us into a blind alley. Recently, many students of obesity have reverted to the nihilistic attitude that obesity is caused simply by overeating and that it can only be cured by under eating.

The Diencephalon or Hypothalamus

For those of us who refused to be discouraged there remained one slight hope. Buried deep down in the massive human brain there is a part which we have in common with all vertebrate animals the so-called diencephalon. It is a very primitive part of the brain and has in man been almost smothered by the huge masses of nervous tissue with which we think, reason and voluntarily move our body. The diencephalon is the part from which the central nervous system controls all the automatic animal functions of the body, such as breathing, the heart beat, digestion, sleep, sex, the urinary system, the autonomous or vegetative nervous system and via the pituitary the whole interplay of the endocrine glands.

It was therefore not unreasonable to suppose that the complex operation of storing and issuing fuel to the body might also be controlled by the diencephalon. It has long been known that the content of sugar - another form of fuel - in the blood depends on a certain nervous center in the diencephalon. When this center is destroyed in laboratory animals, they develop a condition rather similar to human stable diabetes. It has also long been known that the destruction of another diencephalic center produces a voracious appetite and a rapid gain in weight in animals which never get fat spontaneously.

The Fat-bank

Assuming that in man such a center controlling the movement of fat does exist, its function would have to be much like that of a bank. When the body assimilates from the intestinal tract more fuel than it needs at the moment, this surplus is deposited in what may be compared with a current account. Out of this account it can always be withdrawn as required. All normal fat reserves are in such a current account, and it is probable that a diencephalic center manages the deposits and withdrawals.

---

[4] There is some clinical evidence to suggest that those symptoms of Cushing's Syndrome which resemble true obesity are caused by the same mechanism which causes common obesity, while the other symptoms of the syndrome are directly due to adrenocortical dysfunction.

When now, for reasons which will be discussed later, the deposits grow rapidly while small withdrawals become more frequent, a point may be reached which goes beyond the diencephalon's banking capacity. Just as a banker might suggest to a wealthy client that instead of accumulating a large and unmanageable current account he should invest his surplus capital, the body appears to establish a fixed deposit into which all surplus funds go but from which they can no longer be withdrawn by the procedure used in a current account. In this way the diencephalic "fat-bank" frees itself from all work which goes beyond its normal banking capacity. The onset of obesity dates from the moment the diencephalon adopts this labor-saving ruse. Once a fixed deposit has been established the normal fat reserves are held at a minimum, while every available surplus is locked away in the fixed deposit and is therefore taken out of normal circulation.

THREE BASIC CAUSES OF OBESITY:

The Inherited Factor

Assuming that there is a limit to the diencephalon's fat banking capacity, it follows that there are three basic ways in which obesity can become manifest. The first is that the fat-banking capacity is abnormally low from birth. Such a congenitally low diencephalic capacity would then represent the inherited factor in obesity. When this abnormal trait is markedly present, obesity will develop at an early age in spite of normal feeding; this could explain why among brothers and sisters eating the same food at the same table some become obese and others do not.

Other Diencephalic Disorders

The second way in which obesity can become established is the lowering of a previously normal fat-banking capacity owing to some other diencephalic disorder. It seems to be a general rule that when one of the many diencephalic centers is particularly overtaxed; it tries to increase its capacity at the expense of other centers.

In the menopause and after castration the hormones previously produced in the sex-glands no longer circulate in the body. In the presence of normally functioning sex-glands their hormones act as a brake on the secretion of the sex-gland stimulating hormones of the anterior pituitary. When this brake is removed the anterior pituitary enormously increases its output of these sex-gland stimulating hormones, though they are now no longer effective. In the absence of any response from the non-functioning or missing sex glands, there is nothing to stop the anterior pituitary from producing more and more of these hormones. This situation causes an excessive strain on the diencephalic center which controls the function of the anterior pituitary. In order to cope with this additional burden the center appears to draw more and more energy away from other centers, such as those concerned with emotional stability, the blood circulation (hot flushes) and other autonomous nervous regulations, particularly also from the not so vitally important fat-bank.

The so-called stable type of diabetes heavily involves the diencephalic blood sugar regulating center. The diencephalon tries to meet this abnormal load by switching energy destined for the fat bank over to the sugar-regulating center, with the result that the fat-banking capacity is reduced to the point at which it is forced to establish a fixed deposit and thus initiate the disorder we call obesity. In this case one would have to consider the diabetes the primary cause of the obesity, but it is also possible that the process is reversed in the sense that a deficient or overworked fat-center draws energy from the sugar-center, in which case the obesity would be the cause of that type of diabetes in which the pancreas is not primarily involved. Finally, it is conceivable that in Cushing's syndrome those symptoms which resemble obesity are entirely due to the withdrawal of energy from the diencephalic fat-bank in order to make it available to the highly disturbed center which governs the anterior pituitary adrenocortical system.

Whether obesity is caused by a marked inherited deficiency of the fat-center or by some entirely different diencephalic regulatory disorder, its insurgence obviously has nothing to do with overeating and in either case obesity is certain to develop regardless of dietary restrictions. In these cases any enforced food deficit is made up from essential fat reserves and normal structural fat, much to the disadvantage of the patient's general health.

The Exhaustion of the Fat-bank

But there is still a third way in which obesity can become established, and that is when a presumably normal fat-center is suddenly -- the emphasis is on suddenly -- called upon to deal with an enormous influx of food far in excess of momentary requirements.

At first glance it does seem that here we have a straight-forward case of overeating being responsible for obesity, but on further analysis it soon becomes clear that the relation of cause and effect is not so simple. In the first place we are merely assuming that the capacity of the fat center is normal while it is possible and even probable that only persons who have some inherited trait in this direction can become obese merely by overeating.

Secondly, in many of these cases the amount of food eaten remains the same and it is only the consumption of fuel which is suddenly decreased, as when an athlete is confined to bed for many weeks with a broken bone or when a man leading a highly active life is suddenly tied to his desk in an office and to television at home. Similarly, when a person, grown up in a cold climate, is transferred to a tropical country and continues to eat as before, he may develop obesity because in the heat far less fuel is required to maintain the normal body temperature.

When a person suffers a long period of privation, be it due to chronic illness, poverty, famine or the exigencies of war, his diencephalic regulations adjust themselves to some extent to the low food intake. When then suddenly these conditions change and he is free to eat all the food he wants, this is liable to overwhelm his fat-regulating center. During the last war[5] about 6000 grossly underfed Polish refugees who had spent harrowing years in Russia were transferred to a camp in India where they were well housed, given normal British army rations and some cash to buy a few extras. Within about three months, 85% were suffering from obesity.

In a person eating coarse and unrefined food, the digestion is slow and only a little nourishment at a time is assimilated from the intestinal tract. When such a person is suddenly able to obtain highly refined foods such as sugar, white flour, butter and oil these are so rapidly digested and assimilated that the rush of incoming fuel which occurs at every meal may eventually overpower the diecenphalic regulatory mechanisms and thus lead to obesity. This is commonly seen in the poor man who suddenly becomes rich enough to buy the more expensive refined foods, though his total caloric intake remains the same or is even less than before.

Psychological Aspects

Much has been written about the psychological aspects of obesity. Among its many functions the diencephalon is also the seat of our primitive animal instincts, and just as in an emergency it can switch energy from one center to another, so it seems to be

---

[5] World War II.

able to transfer pressure from one instinct to another. Thus, a lonely and unhappy person deprived of all emotional comfort and of all instinct gratification except the stilling of hunger and thirst can use these as outlets for pent up instinct pressure and so develop obesity. Yet once that has happened, no amount of psychotherapy or analysis, happiness, company or the gratification of other instincts will correct the condition.

Compulsive Eating

No end of injustice is done to obese patients by accusing them of compulsive eating, which is a form of diverted sex gratification. Most obese patients do not suffer from compulsive eating; they suffer genuine hunger - real, gnawing, torturing hunger - which has nothing whatever to do with compulsive eating. Even their sudden desire for sweets is merely the result of the experience that sweets, pastries and alcohol will most rapidly of all foods allay the pangs of hunger. This has nothing to do with diverted instincts.

On the other hand, compulsive eating does occur in some obese patients, particularly in girls in their late teens or early twenties. Compulsive eating differs fundamentally from the obese patient's greater need for food. It comes on in attacks and is never associated with real hunger, a fact which is readily admitted by the patients. They only feel a feral desire to stuff. Two pounds of chocolates may be devoured in a few minutes; cold, greasy food from the refrigerator, stale bread, leftovers on stacked plates, almost anything edible is crammed down with terrifying speed and ferocity.

I have occasionally been able to watch such an attack without the patient's knowledge, and it is a frightening, ugly spectacle to behold, even if one does realize that mechanisms entirely beyond the patient's control are at work. A careful enquiry into what may have brought on such an attack almost invariably reveals that it is preceded by a strong unresolved sex-stimulation, the higher centers of the brain having blocked primitive diencephalic instinct gratification. The pressure is then let off through another primitive channel, which is oral gratification. In my experience the only thing that will cure this condition is uninhibited sex, a therapeutic procedure which is hardly ever feasible, for if it were, the patient would have adopted it without professional prompting, nor would this in any way correct the associated obesity. It would only raise new and often greater problems if used as a therapeutic measure.

Patients suffering from real compulsive eating are comparatively rare. In my practice they constitute about 1-2%. Treating them for obesity is a heartrending job. They do perfectly well between attacks, but a single bout occurring while under treatment may annul several weeks of therapy. Little wonder that such patients become discouraged. In these cases I have found that psychotherapy may make the patient fully understand the mechanism, but it does nothing to stop it. Perhaps society's growing sexual permissiveness will make compulsive eating even rarer.

Whether a patient is really suffering from compulsive eating or not is hard to decide before treatment because many obese patients think that their desire for food -- to them unmotivated -- is due to compulsive eating, while all the time it is merely a greater need for food. The only way to find out is to treat such patients. Those that suffer from real compulsive eating continue to have such attacks, while those who are not compulsive eaters never get an attack during treatment.

Reluctance to Lose Weight

Some patients are deeply attached to their fat and cannot bear the thought of losing it. If they are intelligent, popular and successful in spite of their handicap, this is a source of pride. Some fat girls look upon their condition as a safeguard against erotic involvements, of which they are afraid. They work out a pattern of life in which their obesity plays a determining role and then become reluctant to upset this pattern and face a new kind of life which will be entirely different after their figure has become normal and often very attractive. They fear that people will like them - or be jealous - on account of their figure rather than be attracted by their intelligence or character only. Some have a feeling that reducing means giving up an almost cherished and intimate part of themselves. In many of these cases psychotherapy can be helpful, as it enables these patients to see the whole situation in the full light of consciousness. An affectionate attachment to abnormal fat is usually seen in patients who became obese in childhood, but this is not necessarily so.

In all other cases the best psychotherapy can do in the usual treatment of obesity is to render the burden of hunger and never-ending dietary restrictions slightly more tolerable. Patients who have successfully established an erotic transfer to their psychiatrist are often better able to bear their suffering as a secret labor of love.

There are thus a large number of ways in which obesity can be initiated, though the disorder itself is always due to the same mechanism, an inadequacy of the diencephalic fat-center and the laying down of abnormally fixed fat deposits in abnormal places. This means that once obesity has become established, it can no more be cured by eliminating those factors which brought it on than a fire can be extinguished by removing the cause of the conflagration. Thus a discussion of the various ways in which obesity can become established is useful from a preventative point of view, but it has no bearing on the treatment of the established condition. The elimination of factors which are clearly hastening the course of the disorder may slow down its progress or even halt it, but they can never correct it.

Not by Weight alone...

Weight alone is not a satisfactory criterion by which to judge whether a person is suffering from the disorder we call obesity or not. Every physician is familiar with the sylphlike lady who enters the consulting room and declares emphatically that she is getting horribly fat and wishes to reduce. Many an honest and sympathetic physician at once concludes that he is dealing with a "nut." If he is busy he will give her short shrift, but if he has time he will weigh her and show her tables to prove that she is actually underweight.

I have never yet seen or heard of such a lady being convinced by either procedure. The reason is that in my experience the lady is nearly always right and the doctor wrong. When such a patient is carefully examined one finds many signs of potential obesity, which is just about to become manifest as overweight. The patient distinctly feels that something is wrong with her, that a subtle change is taking place in her body, and this alarms her.

There are a number of signs and symptoms which are characteristic of obesity. In manifest obesity many and often all these signs and symptoms are present. In latent or just beginning cases some are always found, and it should be a rule that if two or more of the bodily signs are present, the case must be regarded as one that needs immediate help.

Signs and symptoms of obesity

The bodily signs may be divided into such as have developed before puberty, indicating a strong inherited factor, and those which develop at the onset of manifest disorder. Early signs are a disproportionately large size of the two upper front teeth, the first incisor, or a dimple on both sides of the sacral bone just above the buttocks. When the arms are outstretched with the palms upward, the forearms appear sharply angled outward from the upper arms. The same applies to the lower extremities. The patient cannot bring his feet together without the knees overlapping; he is, in fact, knock-kneed.

The beginning accumulation of abnormal fat shows as a little pad just below the nape of the neck, colloquially known as the Duchess' Hump. There is a triangular fatty bulge in front of the armpit when the arm is held against the body. When the skin is stretched by fat rapidly accumulating under it, it may split in the lower layers. When large and fresh, such tears are purple, but later they are transformed into white scar-tissue. Such striation, as it is called, commonly occurs on the abdomen of women during pregnancy, but in obesity it is frequently found on the breasts, the hips and occasionally on the shoulders. In many cases striation is so fine that the small white lines are only just visible. They are always a sure sign of obesity, and though this may be slight at the time of examination such patients can usually remember a period in their childhood when they were excessively chubby.

Another typical sign is a pad of fat on the insides of the knees, a spot where normal fat reserves are never stored. There may be a fold of skin over the pubic area and another fold may stretch round both sides of the chest, where a loose roll of fat can be picked up between two fingers. In the male an excessive accumulation of fat in the breasts is always indicative, while in the female the breast is usually, but not necessarily, large. Obviously excessive fat on the abdomen, the hips, thighs, upper arms, chin and shoulders are characteristic, and it is important to remember that any number of these signs may be present in persons whose weight is statistically normal; particularly if they are dieting on their own with iron determination.

Common clinical symptoms which are indicative only in their association and in the frame of the whole clinical picture are: frequent headaches, rheumatic pains without detectable bony abnormality; a feeling of laziness and lethargy, often both physical and mental and frequently associated with insomnia, the patients saying that all they want is to rest; the frightening feeling of being famished and sometimes weak with hunger two to three hours after a hearty meal and an irresistible yearning for sweets and starchy food which often overcomes the patient quite suddenly and is sometimes substituted by a desire for alcohol; constipation and a spastic or irritable colon are unusually common among the obese, and so are menstrual disorders.

Returning once more to our sylphlike lady, we can say that a combination of some of these symptoms with a few of the typical bodily signs is sufficient evidence to take her case seriously. A human figure, male or female, can only be judged in the nude; any opinion based on the dressed appearance can be quite fantastically wide off the mark, and I feel myself driven to the conclusion that apart from frankly psychotic patients such as cases of anorexia nervosa; a morbid weight fixation does not exist. I have yet to see a patient who continues to complain after the figure has been rendered normal by adequate treatment.

The Emaciated Lady

I remember the case of a lady who was escorted into my consulting room while I was telephoning. She sat down in front of my desk, and when I looked up to greet her I saw the typical picture of advanced emaciation. Her dry skin hung loosely over the bones of her face, her neck was scrawny and collarbones and ribs stuck out from deep hollows. I immediately thought of cancer and decided to which of my colleagues at the hospital I would refer her. Indeed, I felt a little annoyed that my assistant had not explained to her that her case did not fall under my specialty. In answer to my query as to what I could do for her, she replied that she wanted to reduce. I tried to hide my surprise, but she must have noted a fleeting expression, for she smiled and said "I know that you think I'm mad, but just wait." With that she rose and came round to my side of the desk. Jutting out from a tiny waist she had enormous hips and thighs.

By using a technique which will presently be described, the abnormal fat on her hips was transferred to the rest of her body which had been emaciated by months of very severe dieting. At the end of a treatment lasting five weeks, she, a small woman, had lost 8 inches round her hips, while her face looked fresh and florid, the ribs were no longer visible and her weight was the same to the ounce as it had been at the first consultation.

Fat but not Obese

While a person who is statistically underweight may still be suffering from the disorder which causes obesity, it is also possible for a person to be statistically overweight without suffering from obesity. For such persons weight is no problem, as they can gain or lose at will and experience no difficulty in reducing their caloric intake. They are masters of their weight, which the obese are not. Moreover, their excess fat shows no preference for certain typical regions of the body, as does the fat in all cases of obesity. Thus, the decision whether a borderline case is really suffering from obesity or not cannot be made merely by consulting weight tables.

The Treatment Of Obesity

If obesity is always due to one very specific diencephalic deficiency, it follows that the only way to cure it is to correct this deficiency. At first this seemed an utterly hopeless undertaking. The greatest obstacle was that one could hardly hope to correct an inherited trait localized deep inside the brain, and while we did possess a number of drugs whose point of action was believed to be in the diencephalon, none of them had the slightest effect on the fat-center. There was not even a pointer showing a direction in which pharmacological research could move to find a drug that had such a specific action. The closest approach were the appetite-reducing drugs - the amphetamines----- but these cured nothing.

A Curious Observation

Mulling over this depressing situation, I remembered a rather curious observation made many years ago in India. At that time we knew very little about the function of the diencephalon, and my interest centered round the pituitary gland. Froehlich had described cases of extreme obesity and sexual underdevelopment in youths suffering from a new growth of the anterior pituitary lobe, producing what then became known as Froehlich's disease. However, it was very soon discovered that the identical syndrome, though running a less fulminating course, was quite common in patients whose pituitary gland was perfectly normal. These are the so-called "fat boys" with long, slender hands, breasts any flat-chested maiden would be proud to posses, large hips, buttocks and thighs with striation, knock-knees and underdeveloped genitals, often with undescended testicles.

It also became known that in these cases the sex organs could he developed by giving the patients injections of a substance extracted from the urine of pregnant women, it having been shown that when this substance was injected into sexually immature rats it made them precociously mature. The amount of substance which produced this effect in one rat was called one International Unit, and the purified extract was accordingly called "Human Chorionic Gonadotrophin" whereby chorionic signifies that it is produced in the placenta and gonadotropin that its action is sex gland directed.

The usual way of treating "fat boys" with underdeveloped genitals is to inject several hundred International Units twice a week. Human Chorionic Gonadotrophin which we shall henceforth simply call HCG is expensive and as "fat boys" are fairly common among Indians I tried to establish the smallest effective dose. In the course of this study three interesting things emerged. The first was that when fresh pregnancy-urine from the female ward was given in quantities of about 300 cc. by retention enema, as good results could be obtained as by injecting the pure substance. The second was that small daily doses appeared to be just as effective as much larger ones given twice a week. Thirdly, and that is the observation that concerns us here, when such patients were given small daily doses they seemed to lose their ravenous appetite though they neither gained nor lost weight. Strangely enough however, their shape did change. Though they were not restricted in diet, there was a distinct decrease in the circumference of their hips.

Fat on the Move

Remembering this, it occurred to me that the change in shape could only be explained by a movement of fat away from abnormal deposits on the hips, and if that were so there was just a chance that while such fat was in transition it might be available to the body as fuel. This was easy to find out, as in that case, fat on the move would be able to replace food. It should then he possible to keep a "fat boy" on a severely restricted diet without a feeling of hunger, in spite of a rapid loss of weight. When I tried this in typical cases of Froehlich's syndrome, I found that as long as such patients were given small daily doses of HCG they could comfortably go about their usual occupations on a diet of only 500 Calories daily and lose an average of about one pound per day. It was also perfectly evident that only abnormal fat was being consumed, as there were no signs of any depletion of normal fat. Their skin remained fresh and turgid, and gradually their figures became entirely normal, nor did the daily administration of HCG appear to have any side-effects other than beneficial.

From this point it was a small step to try the same method in all other forms of obesity. It took a few hundred cases to establish beyond reasonable doubt that the mechanism operates in exactly the same way and seemingly without exception in every case of obesity. I found that, though most patients were treated in the outpatients department, gross dietary errors rarely occurred. On the contrary, most patients complained that the two meals of 250 Calories each were more than they could manage, as they continually had a feeling of just having had a large meal.

Pregnancy and Obesity

Once this trail was opened, further observations seemed to fall into line. It is, for instance, well known that during pregnancy an obese woman can very easily lose weight. She can drastically reduce her diet without feeling hunger or discomfort and lose weight without in any way harming the child in her womb. It is also surprising to what extent a woman can suffer from pregnancy-vomiting without coming to any real harm.

Pregnancy is an obese woman's one great chance to reduce her excess weight. That she so rarely makes use of this opportunity is due to the erroneous notion, usually fostered by her elder relations, that she now has "two mouths to feed" and must "keep up her strength for the coming event. All modern obstetricians know that this is nonsense and that the more superfluous fat is lost the less difficult will be the confinement, though some still hesitate to prescribe a diet sufficiently low in Calories to bring about a drastic reduction.

A woman may gain weight during pregnancy, but she never becomes obese in the strict sense of the word. Under the influence of the HCG which circulates in enormous quantities in her body during pregnancy, her diencephalic banking capacity seems to be unlimited, and abnormal fixed deposits are never formed. At confinement[6] she is suddenly deprived of HCG, and her diencephalic fat-center reverts to its normal capacity. It is only then that the abnormally accumulated fat is locked away again in a fixed deposit. From that moment on she is suffering from obesity and is subject to all its consequences.

Pregnancy seems to be the only normal human condition in which the diencephalic fat-banking capacity is unlimited. It is only during pregnancy that fixed fat deposits can be transferred back into the normal current account and freely drawn upon to make up for any nutritional deficit. During pregnancy, every ounce of reserve fat is placed at the disposal of the growing fetus. Were this not so, an obese woman, whose normal reserves are already depleted, would have the greatest difficulties in bringing her pregnancy to full term. There is considerable evidence to suggest that it is the HCG produced in large quantities in the placenta which brings about this diencephalic change.

Though we may be able to increase the dieneephalic fat banking capacity by injecting HCG, this does not in itself affect the weight, just as transferring monetary funds from a fixed deposit into a current account does not make a man any poorer; to become poorer it is also necessary that he freely spends the money which thus becomes available. In pregnancy the needs of the growing embryo take care of this to some extent, but in the treatment of obesity there is no embryo, and so a very severe dietary restriction must take its place for the duration of treatment.

Only when the fat which is in transit under the effect of HCG is actually consumed can more fat be withdrawn from the fixed deposits. In pregnancy it would be most undesirable if the fetus were offered ample food only when there is a high influx from the intestinal tract. Ideal nutritional conditions for the fetus can only be achieved when the mother's blood is continually saturated with food, regardless of whether she eats or not, as otherwise a period of starvation might hamper the steady growth of the embryo. It

---

[6] Confinement = the concluding state of pregnancy

seems that HCG brings about this continual saturation of the blood, which is the reason why obese patients under treatment with HCG never feel hungry in spite of their drastically reduced food intake.

The Nature of Human Chorionic Gonadotropin

HCG is never found in the human body except during pregnancy and in those rare cases in which a residue of placental tissue continues to grow in the womb in what is known as a chorionic epithelioma. It is never found in the male. The human type of chorionic gonadotrophin is found only during the pregnancy of women and the great apes. It is produced in enormous quantities, so that during certain phases of her pregnancy a woman may excrete as much as one million International Units per day in her urine - enough to render a million infantile rats precociously mature. Other mammals make use of a different hormone, which can be extracted from their blood serum but not from their urine. Their placenta differs in this and other respects from that of man and the great apes. This animal chorionic gonadotrophin is much less rapidly broken down in the human body than HCG, and it is also less suitable for the treatment of obesity.

As often happens in medicine, much confusion has been caused by giving HCG its name before its true mode of action was understood. It has been explained that gonadotrophin literally means a sex-gland directed substance or hormone, and this is quite misleading. It dates from the early days when it was first found that HCG is able to render infantile sex glands mature, whereby it was entirely overlooked that it has no stimulating effect whatsoever on normally developed and normally functioning sex-glands. No amount of HCG is ever able to increase a normal sex function; it can only improve an abnormal one and in the young hasten the onset of puberty. However, this is no direct effect. HCG acts exclusively at a diencephalic level and there brings about a considerable increase in the functional capacity of all those centers which are working at maximum capacity.

The Real Gonadotrophins

Two hormones known in the female as follicle stimulating hormone (FSH) and corpus luteum stimulating hormone (LSH) are secreted by the anterior lobe of the pituitary gland. These hormones are real gonadotrophins because they directly govern the function of the ovaries. The anterior pituitary is in turn governed by the diencephalon, and so when there is an ovarian deficiency the diencephalic center concerned is hard put to correct matters by increasing the secretion from the anterior pituitary of FSH or LSH, as the case may be. When sexual deficiency is clinically present, this is a sign that the diencephalic center concerned is unable, in spite of maximal exertion, to cope with the demand for anterior pituitary stimulation.[7] When then the administration of HCG increases the functional capacity of the diencephalon, all demands can be fully satisfied and the sex deficiency is corrected.

That this is the true mechanism underlying the presumed gonadotrophic action of HCG is confirmed by the fact that when the pituitary gland of infantile rats is removed before they are given HCG, the latter has no effect on their sex-glands. HCG cannot therefore have a direct sex gland stimulating action like that of the anterior pituitary gonadotrophins, as FSH and LSH are justly called. The latter are entirely different substances from that which can be extracted from pregnancy urine and which, unfortunately, is called chorionic gonadotrophin. It would be no more clumsy, and certainly far more appropriate, if HCG were henceforth called chorionic diencephalotrophin.

HCG no Sex Hormone

It cannot he sufficiently emphasized that HCG is not sex-hormone, that its action is identical in men, women, children and in those cases in which the sex-glands no longer function owing to old age or their surgical removal. The only sexual change it can bring about after puberty is an improvement of a pre-existing deficiency, but never a stimulation beyond the normal. In an indirect way via the anterior pituitary, HCG regulates menstruation and facilitates conception, but it never virilizes a woman or feminizes a man. It neither makes men grow breasts nor does it interfere with their virility, though where this was deficient it may improve it. It never makes women grow a beard or develop a gruff voice. I have stressed this point only for the sake of my lay readers, because, it is our daily experience that when patients hear the word hormone they immediately jump to the conclusion that this must have something to do with the sex-sphere. They are not accustomed as we are, to think thyroid, insulin, cortisone, adrenalin etc, as hormones.

Importance and Potency of HCG

Owing to the fact that HCG has no direct action on any endocrine gland, its enormous importance in pregnancy has been overlooked and its potency underestimated.

---

[7] As we are speaking of purely regulatory disorders, we obviously exclude all such cases in which there are gross organic lesions of the pituitary or of the sex-glands themselves.

Though a pregnant woman can produce as much as one million units per day, we find that the injection of only 125 units per day is ample to reduce weight at the rate of roughly one pound per day, even in a colossus weighing 400 pounds, when associated with a 500- Calorie diet. It is no exaggeration to say that the flooding of the female body with HCG is by far the most spectacular hormonal event in pregnancy. It has an enormous protective importance for mother and child, and I even go so far as to say that no woman, and certainly not an obese one, could carry her pregnancy to term without it.

If I can be forgiven for comparing my fellow-endocrinologists with wicked Godmothers, HCG has certainly been their Cinderella, and I can only romantically hope that its extraordinary effect on abnormal fat will prove to be its Fairy Godmother.

HCG has been known for over half a century. It is the substance which Aschheim and Zondek so brilliantly used to diagnose early pregnancy out of the urine. Apart from that, the only thing it did in the experimental laboratory was to produce precocious rats, and that was not particularly stimulating to further research at a time when much more thrilling endocrinological discoveries were pouring in from all sides, sweeping, HCG into the stiller back waters.

Complicating Disorders

Some complicating disorders are often associated with obesity, and these we must briefly discuss. The most important associated disorders and the ones in which obesity seems to play a precipitating or at least an aggravating role are the following: the stable type of diabetes, gout, rheumatism and arthritis, high blood pressure and hardening of the arteries, coronary disease and cerebral hemorrhage.

Apart from the fact that they are often - though not necessarily - associated with obesity, these disorders have two things in common. In all of them, modern research is becoming more and more inclined to believe that diencephalic regulations play a dominant role in their causation. The other common factor is that they either improve or do not occur during pregnancy. In the latter respect they are joined by many other disorders not necessarily associated with obesity. Such disorders are, for instance, colitis, duodenal or gastric ulcers, certain allergies, psoriasis, loss of hair, brittle fingernails, migraine, etc.

If HCG + diet does in the obese bring about those diencephalic changes which are characteristic of pregnancy, one would expect to see an improvement in all these conditions comparable to that seen in real pregnancy. The administration of HCG does in fact do this in a remarkable way.

Diabetes

In an obese patient suffering from a fairly advanced case of stable diabetes of many years duration in which the blood sugar may range from 3-400 mg%, it is often possible to stop all antidiabetic medication after the first few days of treatment. The blood sugar continues to drop from day to day and often reaches normal values in 2-3 weeks. As in pregnancy, this phenomenon is not observed in the brittle type of diabetes, and as some cases that are predominantly stable may have a small brittle factor in their clinical makeup, all obese diabetics have to be kept under a very careful and expert watch.

A brittle case of diabetes is primarily due to the inability of the pancreas to produce sufficient insulin, while in the stable type, diencephalic regulations seem to be of greater importance. That is possibly the reason why the stable form responds so well to the HCG method of treating obesity, whereas the brittle type does not. Obese patients are generally suffering from the stable type, but a stable type may gradually change into a brittle one, which is usually associated with a loss of weight. Thus, when an obese diabetic finds that he is losing weight without diet or treatment, he should at once have his diabetes expertly attended to. There is some evidence to suggest that the change from stable to brittle is more liable to occur in patients who are taking insulin for their stable diabetes.

Rheumatism

All rheumatic pains, even those associated with demonstrable bony lesions, improve subjectively within a few days of treatment, and often require neither cortisone nor salicylates. Again this is a well known phenomenon in pregnancy, and while under treatment with HCG + diet the effect is no less dramatic. As it does after pregnancy, the pain of deformed joints returns after treatment, but smaller doses of pain-relieving drugs seem able to control it satisfactorily after weight reduction. In any case, the HCG method makes it possible in obese arthritic patients to interrupt prolonged cortisone treatment without a recurrence of pain. This in itself is most welcome, but there is the added advantage that the treatment stimulates the secretion of ACTH in a physiological manner and that this regenerates the adrenal cortex, which is apt to suffer under prolonged cortisone treatment.

Cholesterol

The exact extent to which the blood cholesterol is involved in hardening of the arteries, high blood pressure and coronary disease is not as yet known, but it is now widely admitted that the blood cholesterol level is governed by diencephalic mechanisms. The behavior of circulating cholesterol is therefore of particular interest during the treatment of obesity with HCG. Cholesterol circulates in two forms, which we call free and esterified. Normally these fractions are present in a proportion of about 25% free to 75% esterified cholesterol, and it is the latter fraction which damages the walls of the arteries. In pregnancy this proportion is reversed and it may he taken for granted that arteriosclerosis never gets worse during pregnancy for this very reason.

To my knowledge, the only other condition in which the proportion of free to esterified cholesterol is reversed is during the treatment of obesity with HCG + diet, when exactly the same phenomenon takes place. This seems an important indication of how closely a patient under HCG treatment resembles a pregnant woman in diencephalic behavior.

When the total amount of circulating cholesterol is normal before treatment, this absolute amount is neither significantly increased nor decreased. But when an obese patient with an abnormally high cholesterol and already showing signs of arteriosclerosis is treated with HCG, his blood pressure drops and his coronary circulation seems to improve, and yet his total blood cholesterol may soar to heights never before reached.

At first this greatly alarmed us. But then we saw that the patients came to no harm even if treatment was continued and we found in follow-up examinations undertaken some months after treatment that the cholesterol was much better than it had been before treatment. As the increase is mostly in the form of the not dangerous free cholesterol, we gradually came to welcome the phenomenon. Today we believe that the rise is entirely due to the liberation of recent cholesterol deposits that have not yet undergone calcification in the arterial wall and therefore highly beneficial.

Gout

An identical behavior is found in the blood uric acid level of patients suffering from gout. Predictably such patients get an acute and often severe attack after the first few days of HCG treatment but then remain entirely free of pain, in spite of the fact that their blood uric acid often shows a marked increase which may persist for several months after treatment. Those patients who have regained their normal weight remain free of symptoms regardless of what they eat, while those that require a second course of treatment get another attack of gout as soon as the second course is initiated. We do not yet know what diencephalic mechanisms are involved in gout; possibly emotional factors play a role, and it is worth remembering that the disease does not occur in women of childbearing age. We now give 2 tablets daily of ZYLORIC to all patients who give a history of gout and have a high blood uric acid level. In this way we can completely avoid attacks during treatment.

Blood Pressure

Patients who have brought themselves to the brink of malnutrition by exaggerated dieting, laxatives etc, often have an abnormally low blood pressure. In these cases the blood pressure rises to normal values at the beginning of treatment and then very gradually drops, as it always does in patients with a normal blood pressure. Normal values are always regained a few days after the treatment is over. Of this lowering of the blood pressure during treatment the patients are not aware. When the blood pressure is abnormally high, and provided there are no detectable renal lesions, the pressure drops, as it usually does in pregnancy. The drop is often very rapid, so rapid in fact that it sometimes is advisable to slow down the process with pressure sustaining medication until the circulation has had a few days time to adjust itself to the new situation. On the other hand, among the thousands of cases treated, we have never seen any untoward incident which could be attributed to the rather sudden drop in high blood pressure.

When a woman suffering from high blood pressure becomes pregnant her blood pressure very soon drops, but after her confinement it may gradually rise back to its former level. Similarly, a high blood pressure present before HCG treatment tends to rise again after the treatment is over, though this is not always the case. But the former high levels are rarely reached, and we have gathered the impression that such relapses respond better to orthodox drugs such as Reserpine than before treatment.

Peptic Ulcers

In our cases of obesity with gastric or duodenal ulcers we have noticed a surprising subjective improvement in spite of a diet which would generally be considered most inappropriate for an ulcer patient. Here, too, there is a similarity with pregnancy, in which peptic ulcers hardly ever occur. However we have seen two cases with a previous history

96

of several hemorrhages in which a bleeding occurred within 2 weeks of the end of treatment.

Psoriasis, Fingernails, Hair, Varicose Ulcers

As in pregnancy, psoriasis greatly improves during treatment but may relapse when the treatment is over. Most patients spontaneously report a marked improvement in the condition of brittle fingernails. The loss of hair not infrequently associated with obesity is temporarily arrested, though in very rare cases an increased loss of hair has been reported. I remember a case in which a patient developed a patchy baldness - so called alopecia areata - after a severe emotional shock, just before she was about to start an HCG treatment. Our dermatologist diagnosed the case as a particularly severe one, predicting that all the hair would be lost. He counseled against the reducing treatment, but in view of my previous experience and as the patient was very anxious not to postpone reducing, I discussed the matter with the dermatologist and it was agreed that, having fully acquainted the patient with the situation, the treatment should be started. During the treatment, which lasted four weeks, the further development of the bald patches was almost, if not quite, arrested; however, within a week of having finished the course of HCG, all the remaining hair fell out as predicted by the dermatologist. The interesting point is that the treatment was able to postpone this result but not to prevent it. The patient has now grown a new shock of hair of which she is justly proud.

In obese patients with large varicose ulcers we were surprised to find that these ulcers heal rapidly under treatment with HCG. We have since treated non obese patients suffering from varicose ulcers with daily injections of HCG on normal diet with equally good results.

The "Pregnant" Male

When a male patient hears that he is about to be put into a condition which in some respects resembles pregnancy, he is usually shocked and horrified. The physician must therefore carefully explain that this does not mean that he will be feminized and that HCG in no way interferes with his sex. He must be made to understand that in the interest of the propagation of the species nature provides for a perfect functioning of the regulatory headquarters in the diencephalon during pregnancy and that we are merely using this natural safeguard as a means of correcting the diencephalic disorder which is responsible for his overweight.

TECHNIQUE

Warnings

I must warn the lay reader that what follows is mainly for the treating physician and most certainly not a do-it-yourself primer. Many of the expressions used mean something entirely different to a qualified doctor than that which their common use implies, and only a physician can correctly interpret the symptoms which may arise during treatment. Any patient who thinks he can reduce by taking a few "shots" and eating less is not only sure to be disappointed but may be heading for serious trouble. The benefit the patient can derive from reading this part of the book is a fuller realization of how very important it is for him to follow to the letter his physician's instructions.

In treating obesity with the HCG + diet method we are handling what is perhaps the most complex organ in the human body. The diencephalon's functional equilibrium is delicately poised, so that whatever happens in one part has repercussions in others. In obesity this balance is out of kilter and can only be restored if the technique I am about to describe is followed implicitly. Even seemingly insignificant deviations, particularly those that at first sight seem to be an improvement, are very liable to produce most disappointing results and even annul the effect completely. For instance, if the diet is increased from 500 to 600 or 700 Calories, the loss of weight is quite unsatisfactory. If the daily dose of HCG is raised to 200 or more units daily its action often appears to be reversed, possibly because larger doses evoke diencephalic counter-regulations. On the other hand, the diencephalon is an extremely robust organ in spite of its unbelievable intricacy. From an evolutionary point of view it is one of the oldest organs in our body and its evolutionary history dates back more than 500 million years. This has tendered it extraordinarily adaptable to all natural exigencies, and that is one of the main reasons why the human species was able to evolve. What its evolution did not prepare it for were the conditions to which human culture and civilization now expose it.

History taking

When a patient first presents himself for treatment, we take a general history and note the time when the first signs of overweight were observed. We try to establish the highest weight the patient has ever had in his life (obviously excluding pregnancy), when this was, and what measures have hitherto been taken in an effort to reduce.

It has been our experience that those patients who have been taking thyroid preparations for long periods have a slightly lower average loss of weight under treatment with HCG than those who have never taken thyroid. This is even so in those patients who have been taking thyroid because they had an abnormally low basal metabolic rate. In many of these cases the low BMR is not due to any intrinsic deficiency of the thyroid gland, but rather to a lack of diencephalic stimulation of the thyroid gland via the anterior pituitary lobe. We never allow thyroid to be taken during treatment, and yet a BMR which was very low before treatment is usually found to be normal after a week or two of HCG + diet. Needless to say, this does not apply to those cases in which a thyroid deficiency has been produced by the surgical removal of a part of an overactive gland. It is also most important to ascertain whether the patient has taken diuretics (water eliminating pills) as this also decreases the weight loss under the HCG regimen.

Returning to our procedure, we next ask the patient a few questions to which he is held to reply simply with "yes" or "no". These questions are: Do you suffer from headaches? rheumatic pains? menstrual disorders? constipation? breathlessness or exertion? swollen ankles? Do you consider yourself greedy? Do you feel the need to eat snacks between meals?

The patient then strips and is weighed and measured. The normal weight for his height, age, skeletal and muscular build is established from tables of statistical averages, whereby in women it is often necessary to make an allowance for particularly large and heavy breasts. The degree of overweight is then calculated, and from this the duration of treatment can be roughly assessed on the basis of an average loss of weight of a little less than a pound, say 300-400 grams-per injection, per day. It is a particularly interesting feature of the HCG treatment that in reasonably cooperative patients this figure is remarkably constant, regardless of sex, age and degree of overweight.

The Duration of Treatment

Patients who need to lose 15 pounds (7 kg.) or less require 26 days treatment with 23 daily injections. The extra three days are needed because all patients must continue the 500-Calorie diet for three days after the last injection. This is a very essential part of the treatment, because if they start eating normally as long as there is even a trace of HCG in their body they put on weight alarmingly at the end of the treatment. After three days when all the HCG has been eliminated this does not happen, because the blood is then no longer saturated with food and can thus accommodate an extra influx from the intestines without increasing its volume by retaining water.

We never give a treatment lasting less than 26 days, even in patients needing to lose only 5 pounds. It seems that even in the mildest cases of obesity the diencephalon requires about three
weeks rest from the maximal exertion to which it has been previously subjected in order to regain fully its normal fat-banking capacity. Clinically this expresses itself, in the fact that, when in these mild cases, treatment is stopped as soon as the weight is normal,

which may be achieved in a week, it is much more easily regained than after a full course of 23 injections.

As soon as such patients have lost all their abnormal superfluous fat, they at once begin to feel ravenously hungry in spite of continued injections. This is because HCG only puts abnormal fat into circulation and cannot, in the doses used, liberate normal fat deposits; indeed, it seems to prevent their consumption. As soon as their statistically normal weight is reached, these patients are put on 800-1000 Calories for the rest of the treatment. The

diet is arranged in such a way that the weight remains perfectly stationary and is thus continued for three days after the 23rd injection. Only then are the patients free to eat anything they please except sugar and starches for the next three weeks.

Such early cases are common among actresses, models, and persons who are tired of obesity, having seen its ravages in other members of their family. Film actresses frequently explain that they must weigh less than normal. With this request we flatly refuse to comply, first, because we undertake to cure a disorder, not to create a new one, and second, because it is in the nature of the HCG method that it is self limiting. It becomes completely ineffective as soon as all abnormal fat is consumed. Actresses with a slight tendency to obesity, having tried all manner of reducing methods, invariably come to the conclusion that their figure is satisfactory only when they are underweight, simply because none of these methods remove their superfluous fat deposits. When they see that under HCG their figure improves out of all proportion to the amount of weight lost, they are nearly always content to remain within their normal weight-range.

When a patient has more than 15 pounds to lose the treatment takes longer but the maximum we give in a single course is 40 injections, nor do we as a rule allow patients to lose more than 34 lbs. (15 Kg.) at a time. The treatment is stopped when either 34 lbs. have been lost or 40 injections have been given. The only exception we make is in the case of grotesquely obese patients who may be allowed to lose an additional 5-6 lbs. if this occurs before the 40 injections are up.

Immunity to HCG

The reason for limiting a course to 40 injections is that by then some patients may begin to show signs of HCG immunity. Though this phenomenon is well known, we cannot as yet define the underlying mechanism. Maybe after a certain length of time the body learns to break down and eliminate HCG very rapidly, or possibly prolonged treatment leads to some sort of counter-regulation which annuls the diencephalic effect.

After 40 daily injections it takes about six weeks before this so called immunity is lost and HCG again becomes fully effective. Usually after about 40 injections patients may feel the onset of immunity as hunger which was previously absent. In those comparatively rare cases in which signs of immunity develop before the full course of 40 injections has been completed-say at the

35th injection- treatment must be stopped at once, because if it is continued the patients begin to look weary and drawn, feel weak and hungry and any further loss of weight achieved is then always at the expense of normal fat. This is not only undesirable, but normal fat is also instantly regained as soon as the patient is returned to a free diet.

Patients who need only 23 injections may be injected daily, including Sundays, as they never develop immunity. In those that take 40 injections the onset of immunity can be delayed if they are given only six injections a week, leaving out Sundays or any other day they choose, provided that it is always the same day. On the days on which they do not receive the injections they usually feel a slight sensation of hunger. At first we thought that this might be purely psychological, but we found that when normal saline is injected without the patient's knowledge the same phenomenon occurs.

Menstruation

During menstruation no injections are given, but the diet is continued and causes no hardship; yet as soon as the menstruation is over, the patients become extremely hungry unless the injections are resumed at once. It is very impressive to see the suffering of a woman who has continued her diet for a day or two beyond the end of the period without coming for her injection and then to hear the next day that all hunger ceased within a few hours after the injection and to see her once again content, florid and cheerful. While on the question of menstruation it must he added that in teenaged girls the period may in some rare cases be delayed and exceptionally stop altogether. If then later this is artificially induced some weight may be regained.

Further Courses

Patients requiring the loss of more than 34 lbs. must have a second or even more courses. A second course can be started after an interval of not less than six weeks, though the pause can be more than six weeks. When a third, fourth or even fifth course is necessary, the interval between courses should be made progressively longer. Between a second and third course eight weeks should elapse, between a third and fourth course twelve weeks, between a fourth and fifth course twenty weeks and between a fifth and sixth course six months. In this way it is possible to bring about a weight reduction of 100 lbs. and more if required without the least hardship to the patient.

In general, men do slightly better than women and often reach a somewhat higher average daily loss. Very advanced cases do a little better than early ones, but it is a remarkable fact that this difference is only just statistically significant.

Conditions that must be accepted before treatment

On the basis of these data the probable duration of treatment can he calculated with considerable accuracy, and this is explained to the patient. It is made clear to him that during the course of treatment he must attend the clinic daily to be weighed, injected and generally checked. All patients that live in Rome or have resident friends or relations with whom they can stay are treated as out-patients, but patients coming from abroad must stay in the hospital, as no hotel or restaurant can be relied upon to prepare the diet with sufficient accuracy. These patients have their meals, sleep, and attend the clinic in the hospital, but are otherwise free to spend their time as they please in the city and its surroundings sightseeing, bathing or theater-going.

It is also made clear that between courses the patient gets no treatment and is free to eat anything he pleases except starches and sugar during the first 3 weeks. It is impressed upon him that he will have to follow the prescribed diet to the letter and that after the first three days this will cost him no effort, as he will feel no hunger and may indeed have difficulty in getting down the 500 Calories which he will be given. If these conditions are not acceptable the case is refused, as any compromise or half measure is bound to prove utterly disappointing to patient and physician alike and is a waste of time and energy.

Though a patient can only consider himself really cured when he has been reduced to his statistically normal weight, we do not insist that he commit himself to that extent. Even a partial loss of overweight is highly beneficial, and it is our experience that once a patient has completed a first course he is so enthusiastic about the ease with which the - to him surprising - results are achieved that he almost invariably comes back for more. There certainly can be no doubt that in my clinic more time is spent on damping over-enthusiasm than on insisting that the rules of the treatment be observed.

Examining the patient

Only when agreement is reached on the points so far discussed do we proceed with the examination of the patient. A note is made of the size of the first upper incisor, of a pad of fat on the nape of the neck, at the axilla and on the inside of the knees. The presence of striation, a suprapubic fold, a thoracic fold, angulation of elbow and knee joint, breast-development in men and women, edema of the ankles and the state of genital development in the male are noted.

Wherever this seems indicated we X-ray the sella turcica, as the bony capsule which contains the pituitary gland is called, measure the basal metabolic rate, X-ray the chest and take an electrocardiogram. We do a blood-count and a sedimentation rate and estimate uric acid, cholesterol, iodine and sugar in the fasting blood.

Gain before Loss

Patients whose general condition is low, owing to excessive previous dieting, must eat to capacity for about one week before starting treatment, regardless of how much weight they may gain in the process. One cannot keep a patient comfortably on 500 Calories unless his normal fat reserves are reasonably well stocked. **It is for this reason also that every case, even those that are actually gaining must eat to capacity of the most fattening food they can get down until they have had the third injection**. It is a fundamental mistake to put a patient on 500 Calories as soon as the injections are started, as it seems to take about three injections before abnormally deposited fat begins to circulate and thus become available.

We distinguish between the first three injections, which we call "non-effective" as far as the loss of weight is concerned, and the subsequent injections given while the patient is dieting, which we call "effective". The average loss of weight is calculated on the number of effective injections and from the weight reached on the day of the third injection which may be well above what it was two days earlier when the first injection was given.

Most patients who have been struggling with diets for years and know how rapidly they gain if they let themselves go are very hard to convince of the absolute necessity of gorging for at least two days, and yet this must he insisted upon categorically if the further course of treatment is to run smoothly. Those patients who have to be put on forced feeding for a week before starting the injections usually gain weight rapidly - four to six pounds in 24 hours is not unusual - but after a day or two this rapid gain generally levels off. In any case, the whole gain is usually lost in the first 48 hours of dieting. It is necessary to proceed in this manner because the gain re-stocks the depleted normal reserves, whereas the subsequent loss is from the abnormal deposits only.

Patients in a satisfactory general condition and those who have not just previously restricted their diet start forced feeding on the day of the first injection. Some patents say that they can no longer overeat because their stomach has shrunk after years of restrictions. While we know that no stomach ever shrinks, we compromise by insisting that they eat frequently of highly concentrated foods such as milk chocolate, pastries with whipped cream sugar, fried meats (particularly pork), eggs and bacon, mayonnaise, bread with thick butter and jam, etc. The time and trouble spent on pressing this point upon incredulous or reluctant patients is always amply rewarded afterwards by the complete absence of those difficulties which patients who have disregarded these instructions are liable to experience.

During the two days of forced feeding from the first to the third injection - many patients are surprised that contrary to their previous experience they do not gain weight and some even lose. The explanation is that in these cases there is a compensatory flow of urine, which drains excessive water from the body. To some extent this seems to be a direct action of HCG, but it may also be due to a higher protein intake, as we know that a protein-deficient diet makes the body retain water.

Starting treatment

In menstruating women, the best time to start treatment is immediately after a period. Treatment may also be started later, but it is advisable to have at least ten days in hand before the onset of the next period. Similarly, the end of a course of HCG should never be made to coincide with menstruation. If things should happen to work out that way, it is better to give the last injection three days before the expected date of the menses so that a normal diet can he resumed at onset. Alternatively, at least three injections should be given after the period, followed by the usual three days of dieting. This rule need not be observed in such patients who have reached their normal weight before the end of treatment and are already on a higher caloric diet.

Patients who require more than the minimum of 23 injections and who therefore skip one day a week in order to postpone immunity to HCG cannot have their third injections on the day before the interval. Thus if it is decided to skip Sundays, the treatment can be started on any day of the week except Thursdays. Supposing they start on Thursday, they will have their third injection on Saturday, which is also the day on which they start their 500 Calorie diet. They would then have no injection on the second day of dieting; this exposes them to an unnecessary hardship, as without the injection they will feel particularly hungry. Of course, the difficulty can be overcome by exceptionally injecting them on the first Sunday. If this day falls between the first and second or between the second and third injection, we usually prefer to give the patient the extra day of forced feeding, which the majority rapturously enjoy.

The Diet

The 500 Calorie diet is explained on the day of the second injection to those patients who will be preparing their own food, and it is most important that the person who will actually cook is present - the wife, the mother or the cook, as the case may be. Here in Italy patients are given the following diet sheet.

BREAKFAST: Tea or coffee in any quantity without sugar. Only one tablespoonful of milk allowed in 24 hours. Saccharin or other sweeteners may be used.

LUNCH: 1) 100 grams of veal, beef, chicken breast, fresh white fish, lobster, crab, or shrimp. All visible fat must be carefully removed before cooking, and the meat must be weighed raw. It must be boiled or grilled without additional fat. Salmon, eel, tuna, herring, dried or pickled fish are not allowed. The chicken breast must be removed raw from the bird.

2) One type of vegetable only to be chosen from the following: spinach, chard, chicory, beet-greens, green salad, tomatoes, celery, fennel, onions, red radishes, cucumbers, asparagus, cabbage.

3) One breadstick (grissino) or one Melba toast.

4) An apple or an orange or a handful of strawberries or one-half grapefruit.

DINNER :   The same four choices as lunch.

The juice of one lemon daily is allowed for all purposes. Salt, pepper, vinegar, mustard powder, garlic, sweet basil, parsley, thyme, majoram, etc., may be used for seasoning, but no oil, butter or dressing.

Tea, coffee, plain water, or mineral water are the only drinks allowed, but they may be taken in any quantity and at all times.

In fact, the patient should drink about 2 liters of these fluids per day. Many patients are afraid to drink so much because they fear that this may make them retain more water. This is a wrong notion as the body is more inclined to store water when the intake falls below its normal requirements.

The fruit or the breadstick may be eaten between meals instead of with lunch or dinner, but not more than than four items listed for lunch and dinner may be eaten at one meal.No medicines or cosmetics other than lipstick, eyebrow pencil and powder may be used without special permission

Every item in the list is gone over carefully, continually stressing the point that no variations other than those listed may be introduced. All things not listed are forbidden, and the patient is assured that nothing permissible has been left out. The 100 grams of meat must he scrupulously weighed raw after all visible fat has been removed. To do this accurately the patient must have a letter-scale, as kitchen scales are not sufficiently accurate and the butcher should certainly not be relied upon. Those not uncommon patients who feel that even so little food is too much for them, can omit anything they wish.

There is no objection to breaking up the two meals. For instance having a breadstick and an apple for breakfast or an orange before going to bed, provided they are deducted from the regular meals. The whole daily ration of two breadsticks or two fruits may not be eaten at the same time, nor can any item saved from the previous day be added on the following day. In the beginning patients are advised to check every meal against their diet sheet before starting to eat and not to rely on their memory. It is also worth pointing out that any attempt to observe this diet without HCG will lead to trouble in two to three days. We have had cases in which patients have proudly flaunted their dieting powers in front of their friends without mentioning the fact that they are also receiving treatment with HCG. They let their friends try the same diet, and when this proves to be a failure - as it necessarily must - the patient starts raking in unmerited kudos for superhuman willpower.

It should also be mentioned that two small apples weighing as much as one large one never the less have a higher caloric value and are therefore not allowed though there is no restriction on the size of one apple. Some people do not realize that a tangerine is not an orange and that chicken breast does not mean the breast of any other fowl, nor does it mean a wing or drumstick.

The most tiresome patients are those who start counting Calories and then come up with all manner of ingenious variations which they compile from their little books. When one has spent years of weary research trying to make a diet as attractive as possible without jeopardizing the loss of weight, culinary geniuses who are out to improve their unhappy lot are hard to take.

Making up the Calories

The diet used in conjunction with HCG must not exceed 500 Calories per day, and the way these Calories are made up is of utmost importance. For instance, if a patient drops the apple and eats an extra breadstick instead, he will not be getting more Calories but he will not lose weight. There are a number of foods, particularly fruits and vegetables, which have the same or even lower caloric values than those listed as permissible, and yet we find that they interfere with the regular loss of weight under HCG, presumably owing to the nature of their composition. Pimiento peppers, okra, artichokes and pears are examples of this.

While this diet works satisfactorily in Italy, certain modifications have to be made in other countries. For instance, American beef has almost double the caloric value of South Italian beef, which is not marbled with fat. This marbling is impossible to remove. In America, therefore, low-grade veal should be used for one meal and fish (excluding all those species such as herring, mackerel, tuna, salmon, eel, etc., which have a high fat content, and all dried, smoked or pickled fish), chicken breast, lobster, crawfish, prawns, shrimps, crabmeat or kidneys for the other meal. Where the Italian breadsticks, the so-called grissini, are not available, one Melba toast may be used instead, though they are psychologically less satisfying. A Melba toast has about the same weight as the very porous grissini which is much more to look at and to chew.

In many countries specially prepared unsweetened and low Calorie foods are freely available, and some of these can be tentatively used. When local conditions or the feeding habits of the population make changes necessary it must be borne in mind that the total daily intake must not exceed 500 Calories if the best possible results are to be obtained, that the daily ration should contain 200 grams of fat-free protein and a very small amount of starch.

Just as the daily dose of HCG is the same in all cases, so the same diet proves to be satisfactory for a small elderly lady of leisure or a hard working muscular giant. Under the effect of HCG the obese body is always able to obtain all the Calories it needs from the abnormal fat deposits, regardless of whether it uses up 1500 or 4000 per day. It must be made very clear to the patient that he is living to a far greater extent on the fat which he is losing than on what he eats.

Many patients ask why eggs are not allowed. The contents of two good sized eggs are roughly equivalent to 100 grams of meat, but fortunately the yolk contains a large amount of fat, which is undesirable. Very occasionally we allow egg - boiled, poached or raw - to patients who develop an aversion to meat, but in this case they must add the white of three eggs to the one they eat whole. In countries where cottage cheese made from skimmed milk is available 100 grams may occasionally be used instead of the meat, but no other cheeses are allowed.

Vegetarians

Strict vegetarians such as orthodox Hindus present a special problem, because milk and curds are the only animal protein they will eat. To supply them with sufficient protein of animal origin they must drink 500 cc. of skimmed milk per day, though part of this ration can be taken as curds. As far as fruit, vegetables and starch are concerned, their diet is the same as that of non-vegetarians; they cannot be allowed their usual intake of vegetable proteins from leguminous plants such as beans or from wheat or nuts, nor can they have their customary rice. In spite of these severe restrictions, their average loss is about half that of non-vegetarians, presumably owing to the sugar content of the milk.

Faulty Dieting

Few patients will take one's word for it that the slightest deviation from the diet has under HCG disastrous results as far as the weight is concerned. This extreme sensitivity has the advantage that the smallest error is immediately detectable at the daily weighing but most patients have to make the experience before they will believe it.

Persons in high official positions such as embassy personnel, politicians, senior executives, etc., who are obliged to attend social functions to which they cannot bring their meager meal must be told beforehand that an official dinner will cost them the loss of about three days treatment, however careful they are and in spite of a friendly and would-be cooperative host. We generally advise them to avoid all-round embarrassment, the almost inevitable turn of conversation to their weight problem and the outpouring of lay counsel from their table partners by not letting it be known that they are under treatment. They should take dainty servings of everything, hide what they can under the cutlery and book the gain which may take three days to get rid of as one of the sacrifices which their profession entails. Allowing three days for their correction, such incidents do not jeopardize the treatment, provided they do not occur all too frequently in which case treatment should be postponed to a socially more peaceful season.

Vitamins and Anemia

Sooner or later most patients express a fear that they may be running out of vitamins or that the restricted diet may make them anemic. On this score the physician can confidently relieve their apprehension by explaining that every time they lose a pound of fatty tissue, which they do almost daily, only the actual fat is burned up; all the vitamins, the proteins, the blood, and the minerals which this tissue contains in abundance are fed back into the body. Actually, a low blood count not due to any serious disorder of the blood forming tissues improves during treatment, and we have never encountered a significant protein deficiency nor signs of a lack of vitamins in patients who are dieting regularly.

The First Days of Treatment

On the day of the third injection it is almost routine to hear two remarks. One is: "You know, Doctor, I'm sure it's only psychological, but I already feel quite different". So common is this remark, even from very skeptical patients that we hesitate to accept the psychological interpretation. The other typical remark is: "Now that I have been allowed to eat anything I want, I can't get it down. Since yesterday I feel like a stuffed pig. Food just doesn't seem to interest me any more, and I am longing to get on with your diet". Many patients notice that they are passing more urine and that the swelling in their ankles is less even before they start dieting.

On the day of the fourth injection most patients declare that they are feeling fine. They have usually lost two pounds or more, some say they feel a bit empty but hasten to explain that this does not amount to hunger. Some complain of a mild headache of which they have been forewarned and for which they have been given permission to take aspirin.

During the second and third day of dieting - that is, the fifth and sixth injection- these minor complaints improve while the weight continues to drop at about double the usually overall average of almost one pound per day, so that a moderately severe case may by the fourth day of dieting have lost as much as 8- 10 lbs.

It is usually at this point that a difference appears between those patients who have literally eaten to capacity during the first two days of treatment and those who have not.

The former feel remarkably well; they have no hunger, nor do they feel tempted when others eat normally at the same table. They feel lighter, more clear-headed and notice a desire to move quite contrary to their previous lethargy. Those who have disregarded the advice to eat to capacity continue to have minor discomforts and do not have the same euphoric sense of well-being until about a week later. It seems that their normal fat reserves require that much more time before they are fully stocked.

Fluctuations in weight loss

After the fourth or fifth day of dieting the daily loss of weight begins to decrease to one pound or somewhat less per day, and there is a smaller urinary output. Men often continue to lose regularly at that rate, but women are more irregular in spite of faultless dieting. There may be no drop at all for two or three days and then a sudden loss which reestablishes the normal average. These fluctuations are entirely due to variations in the retention and elimination of water, which are more marked in women than in men.

The weight registered by the scale is determined by two processes not necessarily synchronized. Under the influence of HCG, fat is being extracted from the cells, in which it is stored in the fatty tissue. When these cells are empty and therefore serve no purpose, the body breaks down the cellular structure and absorbs it, but breaking up of useless cells, connective tissue, blood vessels, etc., may lag behind the process of fat-extraction. When this happens the body appears to replace some of the extracted fat with water which is retained for this purpose. As water is heavier than fat the scales may show no loss of weight, although sufficient fat has actually been consumed to make up for the deficit in the 500-Calorie diet. When then such tissue is finally broken down, the water is liberated and there is a sudden flood of urine and a marked loss of weight. This simple interpretation of what is really an extremely complex mechanism is the one we give those patients who want to know why it is that on certain days they do not lose, though they have committed no dietary error.

Patients who have previously regularly used diuretics as a method of reducing, lose fat during the first two or three weeks of treatment which shows in their measurements, but the scale may show little or no loss because they are replacing the normal water content of their body which has been dehydrated. Diuretics should never be used for reducing.

Interruptions of Weight Loss

We distinguish four types of interruption in the regular daily loss. The first is the one that has already been mentioned in which the weight stays stationary for a day or two, and this occurs, particularly towards the end of a course, in almost every case.

The Plateau

The second type of interruption we call a "plateau". A plateau lasts 4-6 days and frequently occurs during the second half of a full course, particularly in patients that have been doing well and whose overall average of nearly a pound per effective injection has been maintained. Those who are losing more than the average all have a plateau sooner or later. A plateau always corrects, itself, but many patients who have become accustomed to a regular daily loss get unnecessarily worried and begin to fret. No amount of explanation convinces them that a plateau does not mean that they are no longer responding normally to treatment.

In such cases we consider it permissible, for purely psychological reasons, to break up the plateau. This can be done in two ways. One is a so-called "apple day". An apple-day begins at lunch and continues until just before lunch of the following day. The patients are given six large apples and are told to eat one whenever they feel the desire though six apples is the maximum allowed. During an apple-day no other food or liquids except plain water are allowed and of water they may only drink just enough to quench an uncomfortable thirst if eating an apple still leaves them thirsty. Most patients feel no need for water and are quite happy with their six apples. Needless to say, an apple-day may never be given on the day on which there is no injection. The apple-day produces a gratifying loss of weight on the following day, chiefly due to the elimination of water. This water is not regained when the patients resume their normal 500-Calorie diet at lunch, and on the following days they continue to lose weight satisfactorily.

The other way to break up a plateau is by giving a non-mercurial diuretic[8] for one day. This is simpler for the patient but we prefer the apple-day as we sometimes find that though the diuretic is very effective on the following day it may take two to three days before the normal daily reduction is resumed, throwing the patient into a new fit of despair. It is useless to give either an apple-day or a diuretic unless the weight has been stationary for at least four days without any dietary error having been committed.

Reaching a Former Level

The third type of interruption in the regular loss of weight may last much longer - ten days to two weeks. Fortunately, it is rare and only occurs in very advanced cases, and then hardly ever during the first course of treatment. It is seen only in those patients who during some period of their lives have maintained a certain fixed degree of obesity for ten years or more and have then at some time rapidly increased beyond that weight. When then in the course of treatment the former level is reached, it may take two weeks of no loss, in spite of HCG and diet, before further reduction is normally resumed.

---

[8] We use 1 tablet of hygroton.

110

Menstrual Interruption

The fourth type of interruption is the one which often occurs a few days before and during the menstrual period and in some women at the time of ovulation. It must also be mentioned that when a woman becomes pregnant during treatment - and this is by no means uncommon - she at once ceases to lose weight. An unexplained arrest of reduction has on several occasions raised our suspicion before the first period was missed. If in such cases, menstruation is delayed, we stop injecting and do a precipitation test five days later. No pregnancy test should be carried out earlier than five days after the last injection, as otherwise the HCG may give a false positive result.

Oral contraceptives may be used during treatment.

Dietary Errors

Any interruption of the normal loss of weight which does not fit perfectly into one of those categories is always due to some possibly very minor dietary error. Similarly, any gain of more than 100 grams is invariably the result of some transgression or mistake, unless it happens on or about the day of ovulation or during the three days preceding the onset of menstruation, in which case it is ignored. In all other cases the reason for the gain must be established at once.

The patient who frankly admits that he has stepped out of his regimen when told that something has gone wrong is no problem. He is always surprised at being found out, because unless he has seen this himself he will not believe that a salted almond, a couple of potato chips, a glass of tomato juice or an extra orange will bring about a definite increase in his weight on the following day.

Very often he wants to know why extra food weighing one ounce should increase his weight by six ounces. We explain this in the following way: Under the influence of HCG the blood is saturated with food and the blood volume has adapted itself so that it can only just accommodate the 500 Calories which come in from the intestinal tract in the course of the day. Any additional income, however little this may be, cannot be accommodated and the blood is therefore forced to increase its volume sufficiently to hold the extra food, which it can only do in a very diluted form. Thus it is not the weight of what is eaten that plays the determining role but rather the amount of water which the body must retain to accommodate this food.

This can be illustrated by mentioning the case of salt. In order to hold one teaspoonful of salt the body requires one liter of water, as it cannot accommodate salt in any higher concentration. Thus, if a person eats one teaspoonfull of salt his weight will go up by more than two pounds as soon as this salt is absorbed from his intestine.

To this explanation many patients reply: Well, if I put on that much every time I eat a little extra, how can I hold my weight after the treatment? It must therefore be made clear that this only happens as long as they are under HCG. When treatment is over, the blood is no longer saturated and can easily accommodate extra food without having to increase its volume. Here again the professional reader will be aware that this interpretation is a simplification of an extremely intricate physiological process which actually accounts for the phenomenon.

Salt and Reducing

While we are on the subject of salt, I can take this opportunity to explain that we make no restriction in the use of salt and insist that the patients drink large quantities of water throughout the treatment. We are out to reduce abnormal fat and are not in the least interested in such illusory weight losses as can be achieved by depriving the body of salt and by desiccating it. Though we allow the free use of salt, the daily amount taken should be roughly the same, as a sudden increase will of course be followed by a corresponding increase in weight as shown by the scale. An increase in the intake of salt is one of the most common causes for an increase in weight from one day to the next. Such an increase can be ignored, provided it is accounted for. It in no way influences the regular loss of fat.

Water

Patients are usually hard to convince that the amount of water they retain has nothing to do with the amount of water they drink. When the body is forced to retain water, it will do this at all costs. If the fluid intake is insufficient to provide all the water required, the body withholds water from the kidneys and the urine becomes scanty and highly concentrated, imposing a certain strain on the kidneys. If that is insufficient, excessive water will be with-drawn from the intestinal tract, with the result that the feces become hard and dry. On the other hand if a patient drinks more than his body requires, the surplus is promptly and easily eliminated. Trying to prevent the body from retaining water by drinking less is therefore not only futile but even harmful.

Constipation

An excess of water keeps the feces soft, and that is very important in the obese, who commonly suffer from constipation and a spastic colon. While a patient is under treatment we never permit the use of any kind of laxative taken by mouth. We explain that owing to the restricted diet it is perfectly satisfactory and normal to have an evacuation of the bowel only once every three to four days and that, provided plenty of

112

fluids are taken, this never leads to any disturbance. Only in those patients who begin to fret after four days do we allow the use of a suppository. Patients who observe this rule find that after treatment they have a perfectly normal bowel action and this delights many of them almost as much as their loss of weight.

Investigating Dietary Errors

When the reason for a slight gain in weight is not immediately evident, it is necessary to investigate further. A patient who is unaware of having committed an error or is unwilling to admit a mistake protests indignantly when told he has done something he ought not to have done. In that atmosphere no fruitful investigation can be conducted; so we calmly explain that we are not accusing him of anything but that we know for certain from our not inconsiderable experience that something has gone wrong and that we must now sit down quietly together and try and find out what it was. Once the patient realizes that it is in his own interest that he play an active and not merely a passive role in this search, the reason for the setback is almost invariably discovered. Having been through hundreds of such sessions, we are nearly always able to distinguish the deliberate liar from the patient who is merely fooling himself or is really unaware of having erred.

Liars and Fools

When we see obese patients there are generally two of us present in order to speed up routine handling. Thus when we have to investigate a rise in weight, a glance is sufficient to make sure that we agree or disagree. If after a few questions we both feel reasonably sure that the patient is deliberately lying, we tell him that this is our opinion and warn him that unless he comes clean we may refuse further treatment. The way he reacts to this furnishes additional proof whether we are on the right track or not we now very rarely make a mistake.

If the patient breaks down and confesses, we melt and are all forgiveness and treatment proceeds. Yet if such performances have to be repeated more than two or three times, we refuse further treatment. This happens in less than 1% of our cases. If the patient is stubborn and will not admit what he has been up to, we usually give him one more chance and continue treatment even though we have been unable to find the reason for his gain. In many such cases there is no repetition, and frequently the patient does then confess a few days later after he has thought things over.

The patient who is fooling himself is the one who has committed some trifling, offense against the rules but who has been able to convince himself that this is of no importance and cannot possibly account for the gain in weight. Women seem particularly prone to getting themselves entangled in such delusions. On the other hand, it does frequently happen that a patient will in the midst of a conversation unthinkingly spear an olive or forget that he has already eaten his breadstick.

A mother preparing food for the family may out of sheer habit forget that she must not taste the sauce to see whether it needs more salt. Sometimes a rich maiden aunt cannot be offended by refusing a cup of tea into which she has put two teaspoons of sugar, thoughtfully remembering the patient's taste from previous occasions. Such incidents are legion and are usually confessed without hesitation, but some patients seem genuinely able to forget these lapses and remember them with a visible shock only after insistent questioning.

In these cases we go carefully over the day. Sometimes the patient has been invited to a meal or gone to a restaurant, naively believing that the food has actually been prepared exactly according to instructions. They will say: "Yes, now that I come to think of it the steak did seem a bit bigger than the one I have at home, and it did taste better; maybe there was a little fat on it, though I specially told them to cut it all away". Sometimes the breadsticks were broken and a few fragments eaten, and "Maybe they were a little more than one". It is not uncommon for patients to place too much reliance on their memory of the diet-sheet and start eating carrots, beans or peas and then to seem genuinely surprised when their attention is called to the fact that these are forbidden, as they have not been listed.

Cosmetics

When no dietary error is elicited we turn to cosmetics. Most women find it hard to believe that fats, oils, creams and ointments applied to the skin are absorbed and interfere with weight reduction by HCG just as if they had been eaten. This almost incredible sensitivity to even such very minor increases in nutritional intake is a peculiar feature of the HCG method. For instance, we find that persons who habitually handle organic fats, such as workers in beauty parlors, masseurs, butchers, etc. never show what we consider a satisfactory loss of weight unless they can avoid fat coming into contact with their skin.

The point is so important that I will illustrate it with two cases. A lady who was cooperating perfectly suddenly increased half a pound. Careful questioning brought nothing to light. She had certainly made no dietary error nor had she used any kind of face cream, and she was already in the menopause. As we felt that we could trust her implicitly, we left the question suspended. Yet just as she was about to leave the consulting room she suddenly stopped, turned and snapped her fingers. "I've got it," she said. This is what had happened : She had bought herself a new set of make-up pots and bottles and, using her fingers, had transferred her large assortment of cosmetics to the new containers in anticipation of the day she would be able to use them again after her treatment.

The other case concerns a man who impressed us as being very conscientious. He was about 20 lbs. overweight but did not lose satisfactorily from the onset of treatment. Again and again we tried to find the reason but with no success, until one day he said:"I never told you this, but I have a glass eye. In fact, I have a whole set of them. I frequently change them, and every time I do that I put a special ointment in my eyesocket.. Do you think that could have anything to do with it?" As we thought just that, we asked him to stop using this ointment, and from that day on his weight-loss was regular.

We are particularly averse to those modern cosmetics which contain hormones, as any interference with endocrine regulations during treatment must be absolutely avoided. Many women whose skin has in the course of years become adjusted to the use of fat containing cosmetics find that their skin gets dry as soon as they stop using them. In such cases we permit the use of plain mineral oil, which has no nutritional value. On the other hand, mineral oil should not be used in preparing the food, first because of its undesirable laxative quality, and second because it absorbs some fat-soluble vitamins, which are then lost in the stool. We do permit the use of lipstick, powder and such lotions as are entirely free of fatty substances. We also allow brilliantine to be used on the hair but it must not be rubbed into the scalp. Obviously sun-tan oil is prohibited.

Many women are horrified when told that for the duration of treatment they cannot use face creams or have facial massages. They fear that this and the loss of weight will ruin their complexion. They can be fully reassured. Under treatment normal fat is restored to the skin, which rapidly becomes fresh and turgid, making the expression much more youthful. This is a characteristic of the HCG method which is a constant source of wonder to patients who have experienced or seen in others the facial ravages produced by the usual methods of reducing. An obese woman of 70 obviously cannot expect to have her pued face reduced to normal without a wrinkle, but it is remarkable how youthful her face remains in spite of her age.

The Voice

Incidentally, another interesting feature of the HCG method is that it does not ruin a singing voice. The typically obese prima donna usually finds that when she tries to reduce, the timbre of her voice is liable to change, and understandably this terrifies her. Under HCG this does not happen; indeed, in many cases the voice improves and the breathing invariably does. We have had many cases of professional singers very carefully controlled by expert voice teachers, and the maestros have been so enthusiastic that they now frequently send us patients.

Other Reasons for a Gain

Apart from diet and cosmetics there can be a few other reasons for a small rise in weight. Some patients unwittingly take chewing gum, throat pastilles, vitamin pills, cough syrups etc., without realizing that the sugar or fats they contain may interfere with a regular loss of weight. Sex hormones or cortisone in its various modern forms must be avoided, though oral contraceptives are permitted. In fact the only self-medication we allow is aspirin for a headache, though headaches almost invariably disappear after a week of treatment, particularly if of the migraine type.

Occasionally we allow a sleeping tablet or a tranquilizer, but patients should be told that while under treatment they need and may get less sleep. For instance, here in Italy where it is customary to sleep during the siesta which lasts from one to four in the afternoon most patients find that though they lie down they are unable to sleep.

We encourage swimming and sun bathing during treatment, but it should be remembered that a severe sunburn always produces a temporary rise in weight, evidently due to water retention. The same may be seen when a patient gets a common cold during treatment. Finally, the weight can temporarily increase - paradoxical though this may sound - after an exceptional physical exertion of long duration leading to a feeling of exhaustion. A game of tennis, a vigorous swim, a run, a ride on horseback or a round of golf do not have this effect; but a long trek, a day of skiing, rowing or cycling or dancing into the small hours usually result in a gain of weight on the following day, unless the patient is in perfect training. In patients coming from abroad, where they always use their cars, we often see this effect after a strenuous day of shopping on foot, sightseeing and visits to galleries and museums. Though the extra muscular effort involved does consume some additional Calories, this appears to be offset by the retention of water which the tired circulation cannot at once eliminate.

Appetite-reducing Drugs

We hardly ever use amphetamines, the appetite-reducing drugs such as Dexedrin, Dexamil, Preludin, etc., as there seems to be no need for them during the HCG treatment. The only time we find them useful is when a patient is, for impelling and unforeseen reasons, obliged to forego the injections for three to four days and yet wishes to continue the diet so that he need not interrupt the course.

Unforeseen Interruptions of Treatment

If an interruption of treatment lasting more than four days is necessary, the patient must increase his diet to at least 800 Calories by adding meat, eggs, cheese, and milk to his diet after the third day, as otherwise he will find himself so hungry and weak that he is unable to go about his usual occupation. If the interval lasts less than two weeks the patient can directly resume injections and the 500-Calorie diet, but if the interruption lasts longer he must again eat normally until he has had his third injection.

When a patient knows beforehand that he will have to travel and be absent for more than four days, it is always better to stop injections three days before he is due to leave so that he can have the three days of strict dieting which are necessary after the last injection at home. This saves him from the almost impossible task of having to arrange the 500 Calorie diet while en route, and he can thus enjoy a much greater dietary freedom from the day of his departure. Interruptions occurring before 20 effective injections have been given are most undesirable, because with less than that number of injections some weight is liable to be regained. After the 20th injection an unavoidable interruption is merely a loss of time.

Muscular Fatigue

Towards the end of a full course, when a good deal of fat has been rapidly lost, some patients complain that lifting a weight or climbing stairs requires a greater muscular effort than before. They feel neither breathlessness nor exhaustion but simply that their muscles have to work harder. This phenomenon, which disappears soon after the end of the treatment, is caused by the removal of abnormal fat deposited between, in, and around the muscles. The removal of this fat makes the muscles too long, and so in order to achieve a certain skeletal movement - say the bending of an arm - the muscles have to perform greater contraction than before. Within a short while the muscle adjusts itself perfectly to the new situation, but under HCG the loss of fat is so rapid that this adjustment cannot keep up with it. Patients often have to be reassured that this does not mean that they are "getting weak". This phenomenon does not occur in patients who regularly take vigorous exercise and continue to do so during treatment.

Massage

I never allow any kind of massage during treatment. It is entirely unnecessary and merely disturbs a very delicate process which is going on in the tissues. Few indeed are the masseurs and masseuses who can resist the temptation to knead and hammer abnormal fat deposits. In the course of rapid reduction it is sometimes possible to pick up a fold of skin which has not yet had time to adjust itself, as it always does under HCG, to the changed figure. This fold contains its normal subcutaneous fat and may be almost an inch thick. It is one of the main objects of the HCG treatment to keep that fat there.

Patients and their masseurs do not always understand this and give this fat a working-over. I have seen such patients who were as black and blue as if they had received a sound thrashing.

In my opinion, massage, thumping, rolling, kneading, and shivering undertaken for the purpose of reducing abnormal fat can do nothing but harm. We once had the honor of treating the proprietress of a high class institution that specialized in such antics. She had the audacity to confess that she was taking our treatment to convince her clients of the efficacy of her methods, which she had found useless in her own case.

How anyone in his right mind is able to believe that fatty tissue can be shifted mechanically or be made to vanish by squeezing is beyond my comprehension. The only effect obtained is severe bruising. The torn tissue then forms scars, and these slowly contract making the fatty tissue even harder and more unyielding.

A lady once consulted us for her most ungainly legs. Large masses of fat bulged over the ankles of her tiny feet, and there were about 40 lbs. too much on her hips and thighs. We assured her that this overweight could be lost and that her ankles would markedly improve in the process. Her treatment progressed most satisfactorily but to our surprise there was no improvement in her ankles. We then discovered that she had for years been taking every kind of mechanical, electric and heat treatment for her legs and that she had made up her mind to resort to plastic surgery if we failed.

Re-examining the fat above her ankles, we found that it was unusually hard. We attributed this to the countless minor injuries inflicted by kneading. These injuries had healed but had left a tough network of connective scar-tissue in which the fat was imprisoned. Ready to try anything, she was put to bed for the remaining three weeks of her first course with her lower legs tightly strapped in unyielding bandages. Every day the pressure was increased. The combination of HCG, diet and strapping brought about a marked improvement in the shape of her ankles. At the end of her first course she returned to her home abroad. Three months later she came back for her second course. She had maintained both her weight and the improvement of her ankles. The same procedure was repeated, and after five weeks she left the hospital with a normal weight and legs that, if not exactly shapely, were at least unobtrusive. Where no such injuries of the tissues have been inflicted by inappropriate methods of treatment, these drastic measures are never necessary.

Blood Sugar

Towards the end of a course or when a patient has nearly reached his normal weight it occasionally happens that the blood sugar drops below normal, and we have even seen this in patients who had an abnormally high blood sugar before treatment. Such an attack of hypoglycemia is almost identical with the one seen in diabetics who have taken too much insulin. The attack comes on suddenly; there is the same feeling of lightheadedness, weakness in the knees, trembling, and unmotivated sweating; but under HCG, hypoglycemia does not produce any feeling of hunger. All these symptoms are almost instantly relieved by taking two heaped teaspoons of sugar.

In the course of treatment the possibility of such an attack is explained to those patients who are in a phase in which a drop in blood sugar may occur. They are instructed to keep sugar or glucose sweets handy, particularly when driving a car. They are also told to watch the effect of taking sugar very carefully and report the following day. This is important, because anxious patients to whom such an attack has been explained are apt to take sugar unnecessarily, in which case it inevitably produces a gain in weight and does not dramatically relieve the symptoms for which it was taken, proving that these were not due to hypoglycemia. Some patients mistake the effects of emotional stress for hypoglycemia. When the symptoms are quickly relieved by sugar this is proof that they were indeed due to an abnormal lowering of the blood sugar, and in that case there is no increase in the weight on the following day. We always suggest that sugar be taken if the patient is in doubt.

Once such an attack has been relieved with sugar we have never seen it recur on the immediately subsequent days, and only very rarely does a patient have two such attacks separated by several days during a course of treatment. In patients who have not eaten sufficiently during the first two days of treatment we sometimes give sugar when the minor symptoms usually felt during the first three days of treatment continue beyond that time, and in some cases this has seemed to speed up the euphoria ordinarily associated with the HCG method.

The Ratio of Pounds to Inches

An interesting feature of the HCG method is that, regardless of how fat a patient is, the greatest circumference -- abdomen or hips as the case may be is reduced at a constant rate which is extraordinarily close to 1 cm. per kilogram of weight lost. At the beginning of treatment the change in measurements is somewhat greater than this, but at the end of a course it is almost invariably found that the girth is as many centimeters less as the number of kilograms by which the weight has been reduced. I have never seen this clear cut relationship in patients that try to reduce by dieting only.

Preparing the Solution

Human chorionic gonadotrophin comes on the market as a highly soluble powder which is the pure substance extracted from the urine of pregnant women. Such preparations are carefully standardized, and any brand made by a reliable pharmaceutical

119

company is probably as good as any other. The substance should be extracted from the urine and not from the placenta, and it must of course be of human and not of animal origin. The powder is sealed in ampoules or in rubber-capped bottles in varying amounts which are stated in International Units. In this form HCG is stable; however, only such preparations should be used that have the date of manufacture and the date of expiry clearly stated on the label or package. A suitable solvent is always supplied in a separate ampoule in the same package.

Once HCG is in solution it is far less stable. It may be kept at room-temperature for two to three days, but if the solution must be kept longer it should always be refrigerated. When treating only one or two cases simultaneously, vials containing a small number of units say 1000 I.U. should be used. The 10 cc. of solvent which is supplied by the manufacturer is injected into the rubber- capped bottle containing the HCG, and the powder must dissolve instantly. Of this solution 1.25 cc. are withdrawn for each injection. One such bottle of 1000 I.U. therefore furnishes 8 injections. When more than one patient is being treated, they should not each have their own bottle but rather all be injected from the same vial and a fresh solution made when this is empty.

As we are usually treating a fair number of patients at the same time, we prefer to use vials containing 5000 units. With these the manufactures also supply 10 cc. of solvent. Of such a solution 0.25 cc. contain the 125 I.U., which is the standard dose for all cases and which should never be exceeded. This small amount is awkward to handle accurately (it requires an insulin syringe) and is wasteful, because there is a loss of solution in the nozzle of the syringe and in the needle. We therefore prefer a higher dilution, which we prepare in the following way: The solvent supplied is injected into the rubbercapped bottle containing the 5000 I.U . As these bottles are too small to hold more solvent, we withdraw 5 cc., inject it into an empty rubber-capped bottle and add 5 cc. of normal saline to each bottle. This gives us 10 cc. of solution in each bottle, and of this solution 0.5 cc. contains 125 I.U. This amount is convenient to inject with an ordinary syringe.

Injecting

HCG produces little or no tissue-reaction, it is completely painless and in the many thousands of injections we have given we have never seen an inflammatory or suppurative reaction at the site of the injection.

One should avoid leaving a vacuum in the bottle after preparing the solution or after withdrawal of the amount required for the injections as otherwise alcohol used for sterilizing a frequently perforated rubber cap might be drawn into the solution. When sharp needles are used, it sometimes happens that a little bit of rubber is punched out of the rubber cap and can be seen as a small black speck floating in the solution. As these bits of rubber are heavier than the solution they rapidly settle out, and it is thus easy to avoid drawing them into the syringe.

We use very fine needles that are two inches long and inject deep intragluteally in the outer upper quadrant of the buttocks. The injection should if possible not be given into the superficial fat layers, which in very obese patients must be compressed so as to enable the needle to reach the muscle. Obviously needles and syringes must be carefully washed, sterilized and handled aseptically.[9] It is also important that the daily injection should be given at intervals as close to 24 hours as possible. Any attempt to economize in time by giving larger doses at longer intervals is doomed to produce less satisfactory results.

There are hardly any contraindications to the HCG method. Treatment can be continued in the presence of abscesses, suppuration, large infected wounds and major fractures. Surgery and general anesthesia are no reason to stop and we have given treatment during a severe attack of malaria. Acne or boils are no contraindication; the former usually clears up, and furunculosis comes to an end. Thrombophlebitis is no contraindication, and we have treated several obese patients with HCG and the 500-Calorie diet while suffering from this condition. Our impression has been that in obese patients the phlebitis does rather better and certainly no worse than under the usual treatment alone. This also applies to patients suffering from varicose ulcers which tend to heal rapidly.

Fibroids

While uterine fibroids seem to be in no way affected by HCG in the doses we use, we have found that very large, externally palpable uterine myomas are apt to give trouble. We are convinced that this is entirely due to the rather sudden disappearance of fat from the pelvic bed upon which they rest and that it is the weight of the tumor pressing on the underlying tissues which accounts for the discomfort or pain which may arise during treatment. While we disregard even fair-sized or multiple myomas, we insist that very large ones be operated before treatment. We have had patients present themselves for reducing fat from their abdomen who showed no signs of obesity, but had a large abdominal tumor.

Gallstones

Small stones in the gall bladder may in patients who have recently had typical colics cause more frequent colics under treatment with HCG. This may be due to the almost complete absence of fat from the diet, which prevents the normal emptying of the

---

[9] NOTE: This practice is obsolete. Modern sanitary methods dictate throwing away used needles and syringes and using new ones for each injection.

gall bladder. Before undertaking treatment we explain to such patients that there is a risk of more frequent and possibly severe symptoms and that it may become necessary to operate. If they are prepared to take this risk and provided they agree to undergo an operation if we consider this imperative, we proceed with treatment, as after weight reduction with HCG the operative risk is considerably reduced in an obese patient. In such cases we always give a drug which stimulates the flow of bile, and in the majority of cases nothing untoward happens. On the other hand, we have looked for and not found any evidence to suggest that the HCG treatment leads to the formation of gallstones as pregnancy sometimes does.

The Heart

Disorders of the heart are not as a rule contraindications. In fact, the removal of abnormal fat - particularly from the heart-muscle and from the surrounding of the coronary arteries - can only be beneficial in cases of myocardial weakness, and many such patients are referred to us by cardiologists. Within the first week of treatment all patients - not only heart cases - remark that they have lost much of their breathlessness

Coronary Occlusion

In obese patients who have recently survived a coronary occlusion, we adopt the following procedure in collaboration with the cardiologist. We wait until no further electrocardiographic changes have occurred for a period of three months. Routine treatment is then started under careful control and it is usual to find a further electrocardiographic improvement of a condition which was previously stationary.

In the thousands of cases we have treated we have not once seen any sort of coronary incident occur during or shortly after treatment. The same applies to cerebral vascular accidents. Nor have we ever seen a case of thrombosis of any sort develop during treatment, even though a high blood pressure is rapidly lowered. In this respect, too, the HCG treatment resembles pregnancy.

Teeth and Vitamins

Patients whose teeth are in poor repair sometimes get more trouble under prolonged treatment, just as may occur in pregnancy. In such cases we do allow calcium and vitamin D, though not in an oily solution. The only other vitamin we permit is vitamin C, which we use in large doses combined with an antihistamine at the onset of a common cold. There is no objection to the use of an antibiotic if this is required, for instance by

the dentist. In cases of bronchial asthma and hay fever we have occasionally resorted to cortisone during treatment and find that triamcinolone is the least likely to interfere with the loss of weight, but many asthmatics improve with HCG alone.

Alcohol

Obese heavy drinkers, even those bordering on alcoholism, often do surprisingly well under HCG and it is exceptional for them to take a drink while under treatment. When they do, they find that a relatively small quantity of alcohol produces intoxication. Such patients say that they do not feel the need to drink. This may in part be due to the euphoria which the treatment produces and in part to the complete absence of the need for quick sustenance from which most obese patients suffer.

Though we have had a few cases that have continued abstinence long after treatment, others relapse as soon as they are back on a normal diet. We have a few "regular customers" who, having once been reduced to their normal weight, start to drink again though watching their weight. Then after some months they purposely overeat in order to gain sufficient weight for another course of HCG which temporarily gets them out of their drinking routine. We do not particularly welcome such cases, but we see no reason for refusing their request.

Tuberculosis

It is interesting that obese patients suffering from inactive pulmonary tuberculosis can be safely treated. We have under very careful control treated patients as early as three months after they were pronounced inactive and have never seen a relapse occur during or shortly after treatment. In fact, we only have one case on our records in which active tuberculosis developed in a young man about one year after a treatment which had lasted three weeks. Earlier X-rays showed a calcified spot from a childhood infection which had not produced clinical symptoms. There was a family history of tuberculosis, and his illness started under adverse conditions which certainly had nothing to do with the treatment. Residual calcifications from an early infection are exceedingly common, and we never consider them a contraindication to treatment.

The Painful Heel

In obese patients who have been trying desperately to keep their weight down by severe dieting, a curious symptom sometimes occurs. They complain of an unbearable pain in their heels which they feel only while standing or walking. As soon as they take the weight off their heels the pain ceases. These cases are the bane of the rheumatologists and orthopedic surgeons who have treated them before they come to us. All the usual investigations are entirely negative, and there is not the slightest response to anti-rheumatic medication or physiotherapy. The pain may be so severe that the patients are obliged to give up their occupation, and they are not infrequently labeled as a case of hysteria. When their heels are carefully examined one finds that the sole is softer than normal and that the heel bone - the calcaneus - can be distinctly felt, which is not the case in a normal foot.

We interpret the condition as a lack of the hard fatty pad on which the calcaneus rests and which protects both the bone and the skin of the sole from pressure. This fat is like a springy cushion which carries the weight of the body. Standing on a heel in which this fat is missing or reduced must obviously be very painful. In their efforts to keep their weight down these patients have consumed this normal structural fat.

Those patients who have a normal or subnormal weight while showing the typically obese fat deposits are made to eat to capacity, often much against their will, for one week. They gain weight rapidly but there is no improvement in the painful heels. They are then started on the routine HCG treatment. Overweight patients are treated immediately. In both cases the pain completely disappears in 10-20 days of dieting, usually around the 15th day of treatment, and so far no case has had a relapse though we have been able to follow up such patients for years.

We are particularly interested in these cases, as they furnish further proof of the contention that HCG + 500 Calories not only removes abnormal fat but actually permits normal fat to be replaced, in spite of the deficient food intake. It is certainly not so that the mere loss of weight reduces the pain, because it frequently disappears before the weight the patient had prior to the period of forced feeding is reached.

The Skeptical Patient

Any doctor who starts using the HCG method for the first time will have considerable difficulty, particularly if he himself is not fully convinced, in making patients believe that they will not feel hungry on 500 Calories and that their face will not collapse. New patients always anticipate the phenomena they know so well from previous treatments and diets and are incredulous when told that these will not occur. We overcome all this by letting new patients spend a little time in the waiting room with older hands, who can always be relied upon to allay these fears with evangelistic zeal, often demonstrating the finer points on their own body.

A waiting-room filled with obese patients who congregate daily is a sort of group therapy. They compare notes and pop back into the waiting room after the consultation to announce the score of the last 24 hours to an enthralled audience. They cross-check on their diets and sometimes confess sins which they try to hide from us, usually with the result that the patient in whom they have confided palpitatingly tattles the whole disgraceful story to us with a "But don't let her know I told you."

Concluding a Course

When the three days of dieting after the last injection are over, the patients are told that they may now eat anything they please, except sugar and starch provided they faithfully observe one simple rule. This rule is that they must have their own portable bathroom-scale always at hand, particularly while traveling. They must without fail weigh themselves every morning as they get out of bed, having first emptied their bladder. If they are in the habit of having breakfast in bed, they must weigh before breakfast.

It takes about 3 weeks before the weight reached at the end of the treatment becomes stable, i.e. does not show violent fluctuations after an occasional excess. During this period patients must realize that the so-called carbohydrates, that is sugar, rice, bread, potatoes, pastries, etc, are by far the most dangerous. If no carbohydrates whatsoever are eaten, fats can be indulged in somewhat more liberally and even small quantities of alcohol, such as a glass of wine with meals, does no harm, but **as soon as fats and starch are combined things are very liable to get out of hand.** This has to be observed very carefully during the first 3 weeks after the treatment is ended otherwise disappointments are almost sure to occur.

Skipping a Meal

As long as their weight stays within two pounds of the weight reached on the day of the last injection, patients should take no notice of any increase but the moment the scale goes beyond two pounds, even if this is only a few ounces, they must on that same day entirely skip breakfast and lunch but take plenty to drink. In the evening they must eat a huge steak with only an apple or a raw tomato. Of course this rule applies only to the morning weight. Ex-obese patients should never check their weight during the day, as there may be wide fluctuations and these are merely alarming and confusing.

It is of utmost importance that the meal is skipped on the same day as the scale registers an increase of more than two pounds and that missing the meals is not postponed until the following day. If a meal is skipped on the day in which a gain is registered in the morning this brings about an immediate drop of often over a pound. But if the skipping of the meal - and skipping means literally skipping, not just having a light meal - is postponed the phenomenon does not occur and several days of strict dieting may be necessary to correct the situation.

Most patients hardly ever need to skip a meal. If they have eaten a heavy lunch they feel no desire to eat their dinner, and in this case no increase takes place. If they keep their weight at the point reached at the end of the treatment, even a heavy dinner does not bring about an increase of two pounds on the next morning and does not therefore call for any special measures. Most patients are surprised how small their appetite has become and yet how much they can eat without gaining weight. They no longer suffer from an abnormal appetite and feel satisfied with much less food than before. In fact, they are usually disappointed that they cannot manage their first normal meal, which they have been planning for weeks.

Losing more Weight

An ex-patient should never gain more than two pounds without immediately correcting this, but it is equally undesirable that more than two lbs. be lost after treatment, because a greater loss is always achieved at the expense of normal fat. Any normal fat that is lost is invariably regained as soon as more food is taken, and it often happens that this rebound overshoots the upper two lbs. limit.

Trouble After Treatment

Two difficulties may be encountered in the immediate post-treatment period. When a patient has consumed all his abnormal fat or, when after a full course, the injection has temporarily lost its efficacy owing to the body having gradually evolved a counter regulation, the patient at once begins to feel much more hungry and even weak. In spite of repeated warnings, some over-enthusiastic patients do not report this. However, in about two days the fact that they are being undernourished becomes visible in their faces, and treatment is then stopped at once. In such cases - and only in such cases - we allow a very slight increase in the diet, such as an extra apple, 150 grams of meat or two or three extra breadsticks during the three days of dieting after the last injection.

When abnormal fat is no longer being put into circulation either because it has been consumed or because immunity has set in, this is always felt by the patient as sudden, intolerable and constant hunger. In this sense, the HCG method is completely self-limiting. With HCG it is impossible to reduce a patient, however enthusiastic, beyond his normal weight. As soon as no more abnormal fat is being issued, the body starts consuming normal fat, and this is always regained as soon as ordinary feeding is resumed. The patient then finds that the 2-3 lbs. he has lost during the last days of treatment are immediately regained. A meal is skipped and maybe a pound is lost. The next day this pound is regained, in spite of a careful watch over the food intake. In a few days a tearful patient is back in the consulting room, convinced that her case is a failure.

All that is happening is that the essential fat lost at the end of the treatment, owing to the patient's reluctance to report a much greater hunger, is being replaced. The weight at which such a patient must stabilize thus lies 2-3 lbs. higher than the weight reached at the end of the treatment. Once this higher basic level is established, further difficulties in controlling the weight at the new point of stabilization hardly arise.

Beware of Over-enthusiasm

The other trouble which is frequently encountered immediately after treatment is again due to over-enthusiasm. Some patients cannot believe that they can eat fairly normally without regaining weight. They disregard the advice to eat anything they please except sugar and starch and want to play safe. They try more or less to continue the 500-Calorie diet on which they felt so well during treatment and make only minor variations, such as replacing the meat with an egg, cheese, or a glass of milk. To their horror they find that in spite of this bravura, their weight goes up. So, following instructions, they skip one meager lunch and at night eat only a little salad and drink a pot of unsweetened tea, becoming increasingly hungry and weak. The next morning they find that they have increased yet another pound. They feel terrible, and even the dreaded swelling of their ankles is back. Normally we check our patients one week after they have been eating freely, but these cases return in a few days. Either their eyes are filled with tears or they angrily imply that when we told them to eat normally we were just fooling them.

Protein deficiency

Here too, the explanation is quite simple. During treatment the patient has been only just above the verge of protein deficiency and has had the advantage of protein being fed back

127

into his system from the breakdown of fatty tissue. Once the treatment is over there is no more HCG in the body and this process no longer takes place. Unless an adequate amount of protein is eaten as soon as the treatment is over, protein deficiency is bound to develop, and this inevitably causes the marked retention of water known as hunger-edema.

The treatment is very simple. The patient is told to eat two eggs for breakfast and a huge steak for lunch and dinner followed by a large helping of cheese and to phone through the weight the next morning. When these instructions are followed a stunned voice is heard to report that two lbs. have vanished overnight, that the ankles are normal but that sleep was disturbed, owing to an extraordinary need to pass large quantities of water. The patient having learned this lesson usually has no further trouble.

Relapses

As a general rule one can say that 60%-70% of our cases experience little or no difficulty in holding their weight permanently. Relapses may be due to negligence in the basic rule of daily weighing. Many patients think that this is unnecessary and that they can judge any increase from the fit of their clothes. Some do not carry their scale with them on a journey as it is cumbersome and takes a big bite out of their luggage-allowance when flying. This is a disastrous mistake, because after a course of HCG as much as 10 lbs. can be regained without any noticeable change in the fit of the clothes. The reason for this is that after treatment newly acquired fat is at first evenly distributed and does not show the former preference for certain parts of the body.

Pregnancy or the menopause may annul the effect of a previous treatment. Women who take treatment during the one year after the last menstruation - that is at the onset of the menopause - do just as well as others, but among them the relapse rate is higher until the menopause is fully established. The period of one year after the last menstruation applies only to women who are not being treated with ovarian hormones. If these are taken, the premenopausal period may be indefinitely prolonged.

Late teenage girls who suffer from attacks of compulsive eating have by far the worst record of all as far as relapses are concerned.

Patients who have once taken the treatment never seem to hesitate to come back for another short course as soon as they notice that their weight is once again getting out of hand. They come quite cheerfully and hopefully, assured that they can be helped again. Repeat courses are often even more satisfactory than the first treatment and have the advantage, as do second courses, that the patient already, knows that he will feel comfortable throughout.

Plan of a Normal Course

125 I.U. of HCG daily (except during menstruation) until 40 injections have been given.

Until 3rd injection forced feeding.

After 3rd injection, 500 Calorie diet to be continued until 72 hours after the last injection.

For the following 3 weeks, all foods allowed except starch and sugar in any form (careful with very sweet fruit).

After 3 weeks, very gradually add starch in small quantities, always controlled by morning weighing.

CONCLUSION

The HCG + diet method can bring relief to every case of obesity, but the method is not simple. It is very time consuming and requires perfect cooperation between physician and patient. Each case must be handled individually, and the physician must have time to answer questions, allay fears and remove misunderstandings. He must also check the patient daily. When something goes wrong he must at once investigate until he finds the reason for any gain that may have occurred. In most cases it is useless to hand the patient a diet-sheet and let the nurse give him a "shot."

The method involves a highly complex bodily mechanism, and even though our theory may be wrong the physician must make himself some sort of picture of what is actually happening; otherwise he will not be able to deal with such difficulties as may arise during treatment.

I must beg those trying the method for the first time to adhere very strictly to the technique and the interpretations here outlined and thus treat a few hundred cases before embarking on experiments of their own, and until then refrain from introducing innovations, however thrilling they may seem. In a new method, innovations or departures from the original technique can only be usefully evaluated against a substantial background of experience with what is at the moment the orthodox procedure.

I have tried to cover all the problems that come to my mind. Yet a bewildering array of new questions keeps arising, and my interpretations are still fluid. In particular, I have never had an opportunity of conducting the laboratory investigations which are so necessary for a theoretical understanding of clinical observations, and I can only hope that those more fortunately placed will in time be able to fill this gap.

The problems of obesity are perhaps not so dramatic as the problems of cancer, or polio, but they often cause life long suffering. How many promising careers have been ruined by excessive fat; how many lives have been shortened. If some way -however cumbersome - can be found to cope effectively with this universal problem of modern civilized man, our world will be a happier place for countless fellow men and women.

GLOSSARY[10]

ACNE . . . Common skin disease in which pimples, often containing pus, appear on face, neck and shoulders.

ACTH . . . Abbreviation for adrenocorticotrophic hormone. One of the many hormones produced by the anterior lobe of the pituitary gland. ACTH controls the outer part, rind or cortex of the adrenal glands. When ACTH is injected it dramatically relieves arthritic pain, but it has many undesirable side effects, among which is a condition similar to severe obesity. ACTH is now usually replaced by cortisone.

ADRENALIN . . . Hormone produced by the inner part of the Adrenals. Among many other functions, adrenalin is concerned with blood pressure, emotional stress, fear and cold.

ADRENALS . . . Endocrine glands. Small bodies situated atop the kidneys and hence also known as suprarenal glands. The adrenals have an outer rind or cortex which produces vitally important hormones, among which are Cortisone similar substances. The adrenal cortex is controlled by ACTH. The inner part of the adrenals, the medulla, secretes adrenalin and is chiefly controlled by the autonomous nervous system.

ADRENOCORTEX... See adrenals.

AMPHETAMINES . . . Synthetic drugs which reduce the awareness of hunger and stimulate mental activity, rendering sleep impossible. When used for the latter two purposes they are dangerously habit-forming. They do not diminish the body's need for food, but merely suppress the perception of that need. The original drug was known as Benzedrine, from which modern variants such as Dexedrine, Dexamil, and Preludin, etc., have been derived. Amphetamines may help an obese patient to prevent a further increase in weight but are unsatisfactory for reducing, as they do not cure the underlying disorder and as their prolonged use may lead to malnutrition and addiction.

ARTERIOSCLEROSIS . . . Hardening of the arterial wall through the calcification of abnormal deposits of a fatlike substance known as cholesterol.

ASCHHIEIM-ZONDEK . . . Authors of a test by which early pregnancy can be diagnosed by injecting a woman's urine into female mice. The HCG present in

---

[10] Wherever unfamiliar terms are used, they will be found in their respective alphabetical place. The lay reader can therefore make his own cross-reference.

pregnancy urine produces certain changes in the vagina of these animals. Many similar tests, using other animals such as rabbits, frogs, etc. have been devised.

ASSIMILATE . . . Absorb digested food from the intestines.

AUTONOMOUS . . . Here used to describe the independent or vegetative nervous system which manages the automatic regulations of the body.

BASAL METABOLISM . . . The body's chemical turnover at complete rest and when fasting. The basal metabolic rate is expressed as the amount of oxygen used up in a given time. The basal metabolic rate (BMR) is controlled by the thyroid gland.

CALORIE . . . The physicist's calorie is the amount of heat required to raise the temperature of 1 cc. of water by 1 degree Centigrade. The dieticiari's Calorie (always written with a capital C) is 1000 times greater. Thus when we speak of a 500 Calorie diet this means that the body is being supplied with as much fuel as would be required to raise the temperature of 500 liters of water by 1 degree Centigrade or 50 liters by 10 degrees. This is quite insufficient to cover the heat and energy requirements of an adult body. In the HCG method the deficit is made up from the abnormal fat-deposits, of which **1 lb. furnishes the body with more than 2000 Calories.** As this is roughly the amount lost every day, a patient under HCG is never short of fuel.

CEREBRAL . . . Of the brain. Cerebral vascular disease is a disorder concerning the blood vessels of the brain, such as cerebral thrombosis or hemorrhage, known as apoplexy or stroke.

CHOLESTEROL . . . A fatlike substance contained in almost every cell of the body. In the blood it exists in two forms, known as free and esterified. The latter form is under certain conditions deposited in the inner lining of the arteries (see arteriosclerosis). No clear and definite relationship between fat intake and cholesterol-level in the blood has yet been established.

CHORIONIC . . . Of the chorion, which is part of the placenta or after-birth. The term chorionic is justly applied to HCG, as this hormone is exclusively produced in the placenta, from where it enters the human mother's blood and is later excreted in her urine.

COMPULSIVE EATING. . . A form of oral gratification with which a repressed sex-instinct is sometimes vicariously relieved. Compulsive eating must not be confused with the real hunger from which most obese patients suffer.

CONGENITAL . . . Any condition which exists at or before birth.

CORONARY ARTERIES . . . Two blood vessels which encircle the heart and supply all the blood required by the heart-muscle.

CORPUS LUTEUM . . . A yellow body which forms in the ovary at the follicle from which an egg has been detached. This body acts as an endocrine gland and plays an important role in menstruation and pregnancy. Its secretion is one of the sex hormones, and it is stimulated by another hormone known as LSH, which stands for luteum stimulating hormones. LSH is produced in the anterior lobe of the pituitary gland. LSH is truly gonadotrophic and must never be confused with HCG, which is a totally different substance, having no direct action on the corpus luteum.

CORTEX . . . Outer covering or rind. The term is applied to the outer part of the adrenals but is also used to describe the gray matter which covers the white matter of the brain.

CORTISONE . . . A synthetic substance which acts like an adrenal hormone. It is today used in the treatment of a large number of illnesses, and several chemical variants have been produced, among which are prednisone and triamcinolone.

CUSHING . . . A great American brain surgeon who described a condition of extreme obesity associated with symptoms of adrenal disorder. Cushing's Syndrome may be caused by organic disease of the pituitary or the adrenal glands but, as was later discovered, it also occurs as a result of excessive ACTH medication.

DIENCEPHALON . . . A primitive and hence very old part of the brain which lies between and under the two large hemispheres. In man the diencephalon (or hypothalamus) is subordinate to the higher brain or cortex, and yet it ultimately controls all that happens inside the body. It regulates all the endocrine glands, the autonomous nervous system, the turnover of fat and sugar. It seems also to be the seat of the primitive animal instincts and is the relay station at which emotions are translated into bodily reactions.

DIURETIC. . . Any substance that increases the flow of urine.

DYSFUNCTION . . . Abnormal functioning of any organ, be this excessive, deficient or in any way altered.

EDEMA . . . An abnormal accumulation of water in the tissues.

ELECTROCARDIOGRAM . . . Tracing of electric phenomena taking place in the heart during each beat. The tracing provides information about the condition and working of the heart which is not otherwise obtainable.

ENDOCRINE . . . We distinguish endocrine and exocrine glands. The former produce hormones, chemical regulators, which they secrete directly into the blood circulation in the gland and from where they are carried all over the body. Examples of endocrine glands are the pituitary, the thyroid and the adrenals.

Exocrine glands produce a visible secretion such as saliva, sweat, urine. There are also glands which are endocrine and exocrine. Examples are the testicles, the prostate and the pancreas, which produces the hormone insulin and digestive ferments which flow from the gland into the intestinal tract. Endocrine glands are closely inter dependent of each other, they are linked to the autonomous nervous system and the diencephalon presides over this whole incredibly complex regulatory system.

EMACIATED . . . Grossly undernourished.

EUPHORIA . . . A feeling of particular physical and mental well being.

FERAL . . . Wild, unrestrained.

FIBROID . . . Any benign new growth of connective tissue. When such a tumor originates from a muscle, it is known as a myoma. The most common seat of myomas is the uterus.

FOLLICLE . . . Any small bodily cyst or sac containing a liquid. Here the term applies to the ovarian cyst in which the egg is formed. The egg is expelled when a ripe follicle bursts and this is known as ovulation (see corpus luteurn).

FSH . . . Abbreviation for follicle-stimulating hormone. FSH is another (see corpus luteum) anterior pituitary hormone which acts directly on the ovarian follicle and is therefore correctly called a gonadotrophin.

GLANDS . . . See endocrine.

GONADOTROPHIN . . . See corpus luteum, follicle and FSH. Gonadotrophic literally means sex gland-directed. FSH, LSH and the equivalent hormones in the male, all produced in the anterior lobe of the pituitary gland, are true gonadotrophins. Unfortunately and confusingly, the term gonadotrophin has also been applied to the placental hormone of pregnancy known as human chorionic gonadotrophin (HCG). This hormone acts on the diencephalon and can only indirectly influence the sex-glands via the anterior lobe of the pituitary.

HCG . . . Abbreviation for human chorionic gonadotrophin

HORMONES . . . See endocrine.

HYPERTENSION . . . High blood pressure.

HYPOGLYCEMIA . . . A condition in which the blood sugar is below normal. It can be relieved by eating sugar.

HYPOPHYSIS . . . Another name for the pituitary gland.

134

HYPOTHESIS . . . A tentative explanation or speculation on how observed facts and isolated scientific data can be brought into an intellectually satisfying relationship of cause and effect. Hypotheses are useful for directing further research, but they are not necessarily an exposition of what is believed to be the truth. Before a hypothesis can advance to the dignity of a theory or a law, it must be confirmed by all future research. As soon as research turns up data which no longer fit the hypothesis, it is immediately abandoned for a better one.

LSH . . . See corpus luteum.

METABOLISM . . . See basal metabolism.

MIGRAINE . . . Severe half-sided headache often associated with vomiting.

MUCOID . . . Slime-like.

MYOCARDIUM . . . The heart-muscle.

MYOMA . . . See fibroid.

MYXEDEMA . . . Accumulation of a mucoid substance in the tissues which occurs in cases of severe primary thyroid deficiency.

NEOLITHIC . . . In the history of human culture we distinguish the Early Stone Age or Paleolithic, the Middle Stone Age or Mesolithic and the New Stone Age or Neolithic period. The Neolithic period started about 8000 years ago when the first attempts at agriculture, pottery and animal domestication made at the end of the Mesolithic period suddenly began to develop rapidly along the road that led to modern civilization.

NORMAL SALINE . . . A low concentration of salt in water equal to the salinity of body fluids.

PHLEBITIS . . . An inflammation of the veins. When a blood-clot forms at the site of the inflammation, we speak of thrombophlebitis.

PITUITARY . . . A very complex endocrine gland which lies at the base of the skull, consisting chiefly of an anterior and a posterior lobe. The pituitary is controlled by the diencephalon, which regulates the anterior lobe by means of hormones which reach it through small blood vessels. The posterior lobe is controlled by nerves which run from the diencephalon into this part of the gland. The anterior lobe secretes many hormones, among which are those that regulate other glands such as the thyroid, the adrenals and the sex glands.

PLACENTA . . . The after-birth. In women, a large and highly complex organ through which the child in the womb receives its nourishment from the mother's body. It is the organ in which HCG is manufactured and then given off into the mother's blood.

PROTEIN . . . The living substance in plant and animal cells. Herbivorous animals can thrive on plant protein alone, but man must have some protein of animal origin (milk, eggs or flesh) to live healthily. When insufficient protein is eaten, the body retains water.

PSORIASIS . . . A skin disease which produces scaly patches. These tend to disappear during pregnancy and during the treatment of obesity by the HCG method.

RENAL . . . Of the kidney.

RESERPINE . . . An Indian drug extensively used in the treatment of high blood pressure and some forms of mental disorder.

RETENTION ENEMA . . . The slow infusion of a liquid into the rectum, from where it is absorbed and not evacuated.

SACRUM . . . A fusion of the lower vertebrate into the large bony mass to which the pelvis is attached.

SEDIMENTATION RATE . . . The speed at which a suspension of red blood cells settles out. A rapid settling out is called a high sedimentation rate and may be indicative of a large number of bodily disorders of pregnancy.

SEXUAL SELECTION . . . A sexual preference for individuals which show certain traits. If this preference or selection goes on generation after generation, more and more individuals showing the trait will appear among the general population. The natural environment has little or nothing to do with this process. Sexual selection therefore differs from natural selection, to which modern man is no longer subject because he changes his environment rather than let the environment change him.

STRIATION . . . Tearing of the lower layers of the skin owing to rapid stretching in obesity or during pregnancy. When first formed striae are dark reddish lines which later change into white scars.

SUPRARENAL GLANDS . . . See adrenals.

SYNDROME . . . A group of symptoms which in their association are characteristic of a particular disorder.

THROMBOPHLEBITIS . . . See phlebitis.

THROMBUS . . . A blood-clot in a blood-vessel.

TRIAMCINOLONE . . . A modern derivative of cortisone.

URIC ACID . . . A product of incomplete protein-breakdown or utilization in the body. When uric acid becomes deposited in the gristle of the joints we speak of gout.

VARICOSE ULCERS . . . Chronic ulceration above the ankles due to varicose veins which interfere with the normal blood circulation in the affected areas.

VEGETATIVE . . . See autonomous.

VERTEBRATE . . . Any animal that has a back-bone.

Literary References to the Use of Chorionic Gonadotrophin In Obesity

THE LANCET

Nov. 6, 1954	Article	Simeons
Nov. 15, 1958	Letter to Editor	Simeons
July 29, 1961	Letter to Editor	Lebon
Dec. 9, 1961	Article	Carne
Dec. 9, 1961	Letter to Editor	Kalina
Jan. 6, 1962	Letter to Editor	Simeons
Nov. 26, 1966	Letter to Editor	Lebon

THE JOURNAL OF THE AMERICAN GERIATRIC SOCIETY

Jan. 1956 Article		Simeons
Oct. 1964 Article		Harris & Warsaw
Feb. 1966	Article	Lebon

THE AMERICAN JOURNAL OF CLINICAL NUTRITION

Sept.-Oct. 1959	Article	Sohar
March 1963	Article	Craig et al.
Sept. 1963	Letter to Editor	Simeons
March 1964	Article	Frank
Sept. 1964	Letter to Editor	Simeons
Feb. 1965	Letter to Editor	Hutton
June 1969	Editorial	Albrink
June 1969	Special Article	Gusman

THE JOURNAL OF PLASTIC SURGERY (British)

April 1962	Article	Lebon

THE SOUTH AFRICAN MEDICAL JOURNAL

Feb 1963 Article		Politzer, Berson & Flaks

BOOKS

A.T.W. SIMEONS

POUNDS AND INCHES Privately printed: obtainable only from A.T.W. Simeons, Salvator Mundi International Hospital, Rome, Italy

VETSUCHT (Netherlands Edition) Wetenschappelijke Uitgeverij, N.V. Amsterdam

MAN'S PRESUMPTUOUS BRAIN Longman's, Green, London

E.P. Dutton, New York (hardback)

Dutton Paperbacks, New York

Made in the USA
Lexington, KY
17 January 2013